...ise for Danielle Ofri's
Singular Intimacies

"...discovered ...could draw a line between being a doctor and being a woman, that she could hate one patient and care deeply about another, that she could battle the medical establishment and even herself, and that despite modern medicine and her belief in the power of intellect, death conquers all. . . . Her longtime best friend, Josh, died of a heart attack, which led her to the book's central realization: that her relationship with her patients is a sacred zone, populated by 'living, breathing, feeling people'—like Josh, and like herself. Know thyself: That's the theme of [this] book."

—Diane Scharper, *The Washington Post*

"Danielle Ofri's *Singular Intimacies: Becoming a Doctor at Bellevue* about the emotional life of doctors and their patients, captivated me so much. . . . In the gripping chapter 'M & M' (morbidity and mortality), she chronicles the medical decisions that ended a patient's life. 'I cried for my belief that intellect conquers all,' she says. . . . It's this marriage of intellect and emotion that makes *Singular Intimacies* read like a deftly crafted and luminously written novel."

—Caroline Leavitt, *The Boston Globe*

"[Ofri's] Candide-like adventures as she advances from third-year medical student to resident are harrowing, poetic . . . she always learns something about herself, medicine, and humanity. . . . Every patient deserves a doctor of Ofri's sensibility, one who recognizes the profound vulnerability of relying on strangers."

—Sharon Lieberman, *The Women's Review of Books*

"It takes courage, drive, and a large heart for a young doctor to find beauty in the teeming masses that daily stream through Bellevue's door. . . . Finding meaning and hope where both are often elusive is the strongest reason to read Ofri's book."

—Chloe Breyer, *Hope* magazine

"Ofri is courageous enough to describe the imperfect world of an urban hospital, to detail her failures and missteps as well as triumphs—and the successes are framed in terms of the patients' recovery. . . . This book is satisfying as a portrait of a brave, intelligent and engaging woman, as a coming-of-age story and as a window into the world of medicine. I recommend it highly."

—Lesley Beck, *The Berkshire Eagle*

"Each of the fifteen chapters in *Singular Intimacies* is a gripping account of the tenuous link between life and death. Together, they tell a story that's not as much about a physician's training as about a healer's birth."

—Barbara Nachman, *The Journal News*

PENGUIN BOOKS

SINGULAR INTIMACIES

Danielle Ofri is an attending physician at Bellevue Hospital and Assistant Professor of Medicine at New York University. She is Editor-in-Chief and co-founder of the *Bellevue Literary Review*, the first literary magazine based in a hospital. Her essays have been published in numerous medical and literary journals and anthologies. One chapter of this book was selected by Stephen Jay Gould for *The Best American Essays*; another essay was chosen by Oliver Sacks for *The Best American Science Writing*. She is also Associate Chief Editor of the award-winning medical textbook, *The Bellevue Guide to Outpatient Medicine*. She lives in New York City with her husband and two children.

Singular
Intimacies

BECOMING A DOCTOR AT BELLEVUE

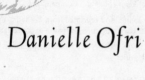

Danielle Ofri

PENGUIN BOOKS

PENGUIN BOOKS

Published by the Penguin Group

Penguin Group (USA) Inc., 375 Hudson Street, New York, New York 10014, U.S.A.

Penguin Books Ltd, 80 Strand, London WC2R 0RL, England

Penguin Books Australia Ltd, 250 Camberwell Road, Camberwell, Victoria 3124, Australia

Penguin Books Canada Ltd, 10 Alcorn Avenue, Toronto, Ontario, Canada M4V 3B2

Penguin Books India (P) Ltd, 11 Community Centre, Panchsheel Park, New Delhi – 110 017, India

Penguin Books (N.Z.) Ltd, Cnr Rosedale and Airborne Roads, Albany, Auckland, New Zealand

Penguin Books (South Africa) (Pty) Ltd, 24 Sturdee Avenue,
    Rosebank, Johannesburg 2196, South Africa

Penguin Books Ltd, Registered Offices: 80 Strand, London WC2R 0RL, England

First published in the United States of America by Beacon Press 2003
Published in Penguin Books 2004

10   9   8   7   6   5   4   3   2   1

Excerpt from "Desert Places" from *The Poetry of Robert Frost* edited by Edward Connery Lathem. Copyright 1936 by Robert Frost © 1964 by Lesley Frost Ballantine, © 1969 by Henry Holt and Company. Reprinted by permission of Henry Holt and Company, LLC.

Excerpt from "Gaudeamus Igitur" by John Stone, reprinted from *Renaming the Streets*, Louisiana State University Press, 1985. Used with the permission of the author.

The names and many distinguishing characteristics of patients mentioned in this work have been changed to protect their identities.

THE LIBRARY OF CONGRESS HAS CATALOGED THE HARDCOVER EDITION AS FOLLOWS:
Ofri, Danielle.
Singular intimacies : becoming a doctor at Bellevue / Danielle Ofri.
p.   cm.
ISBN 0-8070-7252-4 (hc.)
ISBN 0 14 20.0438 3 (pbk.)
1. Ofri, Danielle.   2. Women physicians—United States—Biography.   3. Physicians—United States—
Biography.   4. Women physicians—Training of.   5. Medical history taking—Anecdotes.   I. Title.
    [DNLM: 1. Bellevue Hospital.   2. Clinical Clerkship—Personal Narratives.
3. Medical History Taking—Personal Narratives.   4. Preceptorship—Personal Narratives.
    WB 290 033t 2002]
R692.035   2002
610'.92—dc21   [B]   2002012461

Printed in the United States of America
Designed by Anne Chalmers

FOR THE PATIENTS
OF BELLEVUE
AND FOR JOSH

Contents

Possessing Her Words

"AIR FRANCE," she says. "No other airline. My body must fly to Paris via Air France."

Air France. I write as quickly as I can.

"And they must first go to City Hall to verify the Berneau family name." Her voice warbles through the oxygen mask, direct and dignified, if a bit staccato from her breathlessness.

The anesthesiologist is hovering over Adrienne Berneau with the endotracheal tube and ventilator. Gasping at a rate of thirty-five breaths per minute, with her wispy neck muscles straining like reeds in a summer storm, there isn't much time.

"No ceremony before the interment," she continues in her birdlike voice. "Just a burial at Rue de la Colonnade." I dutifully transcribe her words as the resident physician silences the insistent alarm on the overhead monitors. The anesthesiologist loads his syringe with succinylcholine.

Adrienne Berneau doesn't look sixty-two years old. She has that mythical, ageless beauty that French women seem to possess—her innate charm deceptively triumphant over her Stage IIIB lung cancer.

"Please give my paintings to Pierre Montanier," she says, adjusting the headband that holds her reddish-black hair in place. "And the linens to my neighbor, Sarah Pelnick . . . if she would like them."

"And *you*," she says, looking over her oxygen mask at the intern who is drawing yet another tube of blood, "it is time for *you* to start paying *me* for all that blood I'm giving you." The anesthesiologist draws up

10cc of fentanyl. With no way to be unobtrusive in this crowded and cramped room, the medical student shrinks himself further inside his white lab coat.

I read aloud the words I have transcribed and she is satisfied. With delicate, long-nailed fingers from which many an elegant cigarette has dangled, she signs her name in trembling letters. I add mine as the attending physician directly below. The clerk from Accounts Payable stamps her notary in brusque black ink next to our signatures.

She looks directly at me. "Seven days," she says, swallowing air in quick bites. "*Une semaine.*" Seven days of intubation and treatment is all Adrienne Berneau wants. "If I do not get better," she puffs, "take it out."

Seven days to figure out whether the spidery latticework that has progressed so rapidly on her chest X-ray is an infection or if it is a suffocating return of her cancer. In seven days we could have a reasonable chance of getting an infection under control. But if the biopsy confirms cancer, the seventh day will likely be her last.

We stand in a silent semicircle around her bed and she glances at each of us. "What are you all so nervous about, *mes amis?* We go forward, *non?*" The anesthesiologist flexes the laryngoscope in the air to check that it is functioning properly and it snaps opens with a decisive metallic click.

I hold her hand and ask if she has any further questions. She shakes her head no. On rounds last week I had distributed an article from a medical journal entitled "The Good Death." It talked about how terminally ill patients express a consistent desire to give back to society and so I take a deep breath.

"We train young doctors here," I say, nodding to the medical student, resident, and intern gathered around the bedside in their crisp white coats with pockets bulging from medical paraphernalia. "Is there anything you would like to share with us that would help us all become better doctors?"

She looks around the room, her finely honed cheeks puffing inside the mask. "No, I have no complaints. You have all been my guardian angels."

Heavy swallows and four gazes plummet to the ground.

"Is there anything else we can get you?" I ask, my mouth dry and tentative.

"A clean gown, *s'il vous plaît.* I've made a mess of this one." Four sighs—a request that we can actually fulfill. The respiratory monitor clangs again to warn of dropping oxygen saturation and four arms rush to silence it.

"And you promise me that I sleep through the whole thing? That I do not wake up for the whole week?" I nod, hoping that her low blood pressure won't preclude the use of strong sedatives.

The anesthesiologist raises his eyes to the overhead monitor and then looks to me, parallel lines of wrinkles tensing on his forehead. Three loaded syringes are curled in one hand and the plastic endotracheal tube is clasped in the other.

"Are you ready?" I ask, still holding her hand.

"*Oui.*" Her eyes dart over the edge of the mask, locking us in a tight, airless circle.

"See you later," I say, in the breezy tone I might use with a friend parting ways on the street—and then silently demand to God that we'd better uncover garden variety microorganisms in her lungs and not malignant cells. "We'll see you at the other end." I add, hoping that I am not lying.

I nod to the anesthesiologist as he discharges the first syringe. Adrienne Berneau's sculpted lips with their carefully applied lipstick soften as the sedative whispers through her veins. Then her fingers suddenly tighten around mine in a viselike grip, her nails digging into my palm. I know that it's just the depolarizing effects of the succinylcholine on her muscles, but it feels like a panicked plea for life and I want to shout, "No, don't do it." I want to grab the endotracheal tube from the anesthesiologist's hand to block what may be the beginning of the end. I want to lay my body across hers and protest the silencing of her words. I want to keep her voice with us in this moment, in this room, in this world.

But I know that it can't hold out. Her flailing respiratory muscles and besotted lungs can no longer support this voice that is so much the embodiment of Adrienne Berneau. It will disappear with or without our mechanical intervention. Seven days on the machine is our only chance.

The anesthesiologist lowers the head of the bed and slides the tube down her throat. Her lipstick is smeared in the process. The machine takes over and all at once Adrienne Berneau's body is limp and sallow like every other body lying in wait in the ICU.

One by one I unlock her tensed fingers from mine. The blunt silence is punctuated only by the heaving of the ventilator. Four pairs of eyes catch each other then shudder away in disparate directions. There is the sudden icy awareness that we might be the possessors of Adrienne Berneau's final words. We might be the guardians of her last smile, her final joke, her ultimate *bon mot*. We file out from the room—medical student, intern, resident, and attending physician—our hands dangling awkward and useless, our tears threatening to give way. Like an invisible chain, the silent prayer snakes from one to the next—that maybe Adrienne Berneau will indeed speak again and that we will not be required to carry this burden to our final days.

Seven days we wait.

Seven days we hold her words.

CHAPTER ONE

Drawing Blood

For this is the day you know too little
against the day when you will know too much
John Stone, *"Gaudeamus Igitur"*

ZALMAN WISZHINSKY moaned in his bed. "*Oy,* help me," he wheezed. Sweat accumulated over his bushy white eyebrows as he thrashed about. One arm gripped his chest while the other wormed helplessly in the air. His oxygen mask was filling with condensation, further muffling his Polish accent. He poked his chubby fingers into the side holes of his mask, tugging to dislodge it from his face, but the burly nurse stationed at the head of his bed replaced it firmly and decisively every time. Mrs. Wiszhinsky was fretting about the bedside. "Zalman, *nu,* listen to the doctors." She flung Yiddish admonitions to her husband, who was clearly in no condition to heed them.

After three years of medical school and four years in the laboratory completing a Ph.D., I was at long last "on the wards." My original classmates had already graduated long ago so I didn't know any of the other third-year medical students on my team. Between the vagaries of the schedules of my thesis committee members and the unpredictability of my final experiments, my dissertation defense took place in February. This tossed me onto the wards in March—close to the end of the academic year. The medical student calendar began in July so all the other students on my team already had nearly a year of experience on the medical wards. They knew the difference between an intern, a sub-intern, a resident, and an attending physician. They understood the social distinctions of the various types of white coats. They could discriminate nurses from doctors merely on the basis of the type of stethoscope they carried. They knew where the X-ray department was located. And most impressively, they knew how to draw blood.

Mr. Wiszhinsky had arrived at Bellevue two hours ago; his chief complaint was, "It's not so good today." There wasn't time to take a history from him—everything was happening so fast. His blood pressure was dropping and he was becoming more agitated. The attending (long, neatly tailored white coat; gray hair), residents (long, dirty, nondescript white coats; bags under eyes) and medical students (short, boxy white jackets; overstuffed pockets) scrutinized the monitors. Somebody snapped out, "Page cardiology, *stat!*"

I stood uneasily at the edge of the crowd, squinting in the glare of clinical medicine.

I'd entered Bellevue this morning through the tiny set of double doors that served as the entranceway for this lumbering behemoth of a hospital. Swarms of residents, nurses, patients, and visitors bottlenecked from either direction. The two glass doors were grimy from the thousands of palms that pressed against them each day. The foyer was jammed with white coats and saris, kafiyas and dashikis. Spanish, Tagalog, Bengali, and English elbowed for air space as did the smells of coffee, curry, and homelessness. The doorways were littered with gum wrappers and cigarette butts. Windblown scraps of the *New York Post* and *New York Times* tangled in trampling feet that pressed forward every morning. But these portals led into Bellevue, and now I, too, was in Bellevue, happily part of that swarm pushing through the doors.

A cardiologist materialized with an ultrasound machine and plunked the probe on Mr. Wiszhinsky's chest. The image on the screen was fuzzy, with black specks like an old TV set that needed hangers and crumpled aluminum foil to reign in the reception. I craned my neck to see closer, but there was nothing recognizable in the distorted splotches of gray and white. Knowing grunts and nods, however, came from the crowd around me. They all knew something that I didn't. They all spoke that secret language. Those blurry spots actually had meaning.

Urgent exclamations flew about the room in volleys. "Pericardial effusion!" "Tamponade!" "Cardiogenic shock!" "Page CV surgery, *stat!*" Nurses carted in stainless steel trays overflowing with cryptic gadgets. More white coats arrived, barking orders at one another. Somebody in blue surgical scrubs barreled through the crowd, shoving a medication cart out of his way with one of his muscled biceps, and me out of his way with his other. I retreated out of his path, only to be elbowed by someone else forging a trail to the bedside. I stepped back to avoid further calamity and collided with an irate nurse whose arms were laden with sterile equipment. I struggled to find a place for my ill-adapted body, feeling vaguely like a dinosaur in the age of the mammals.

Charlie, one of the other medical students, took pity on me and translated the scene. Mr. Wiszhinsky had accumulated a large amount of fluid around his heart (pericardial effusion) that was dangerously compressing its chambers (tamponade). His heart could not send enough blood to the rest of his body (cardiogenic shock), so the fluid needed to be drained immediately. "And," he said with a knowing whisper, "this guy should be damn glad he came to a tertiary care hospital like Bellevue. If he'd gone to a crummy little community hospital there's no way he would have gotten all this high-tech stuff and all these experts so quickly. He would've been a goner." I nodded sagely along with Charlie. I didn't know what a tertiary care hospital was, but I was damn glad that we (we!) were one.

Mr. Wiszhinsky was pale and sweaty. Buzzers and alarms squawked from the various accoutrements attached to him. The monitors flashed warning lights in fist-pulsing red. Metal instruments were clanging, people were shouting orders, white coats were jostling—nothing seemed to stand still. Mrs. Wiszhinsky, a wisp of a figure, hovered unsteadily at the edge of the crowd, appearing a bit greenish herself. Several times I saw her open her mouth to ask a question, but she was cut off by the bustle before her lips could even shape a sound. She pulled nervously at her fingers, her husband lost in the crush of bodies and machinery.

There was a fierce argument, apparently between the cardiologists and cardiovascular surgeons, about who should drain the fluid from Mr. Wiszhinsky's heart. I don't know who won the turf battle, but somebody with a receding hairline and a look of authority whipped out a needle that was easily as long as my forearm. The silver spike glistened ominously as he held it up to the light, adjusting the attached syringe. Without a flicker of the bland expression on his face, as though he was about to add detergent to a load of whites, he calmly slammed the needle into Mr. Wiszhinsky's chest. I stared, unable to breath, as the metallic silver sank right through the skin into all those organs that I had learned about so many years ago in anatomy. Important organs! Ones that probably weren't supposed to have needles piercing into them. But suddenly, hazy fluid began to creep into the belly of the syringe. Torpid droplets coalesced into a murky column. The doctor's grip strained against the syringe as the column elongated sluggishly. The fluid resisted the human force with a languid petulance, threatening to suck back into Mr. Wiszhinsky's chest with even the slightest letup of the doctor's pull.

Mr. Wiszhinsky flailed about while the oleaginous fluid was wrung from his heart and the nurses struggled to restrain him. Linda, the senior resident, called out readings from the overhead monitor like an announcer at the races. The junior resident was injecting intravenous medications. The intern ran the EKG machine. The sub-intern was drawing blood samples. Charlie was handing off blood tubes. The head nurse was madly charting every action that transpired. The janitor was cleaning the gauze and iodine that spilled onto the floor.

Everybody had an indispensable role, except me. I prayed fervently that somebody would assign me a task to do, anything at all, no matter how menial. But everyone was busy applying their productive skills for the betterment of humanity. What could I possibly offer? Four years of biochemistry training, a few medical school courses way back, basic history-taking skills from my behavioral science class . . . that was all. What was I doing in this world of medicine, in this world of real people living and dying? How could I possibly deserve to enter those doors of Bellevue, to be part of this tertiary care hospital (thank goodness we were a tertiary care hospital) if I was such an inept dolt? Yes, that's what I was—a drain upon society, the dregs of the system, the type that totalitarian societies deem unworthy of existence and relocate to Siberia. I wished someone would just banish me from civilization this very moment and spare me the humiliation of being so utterly useless.

I had been relegated to the foot of the bed, somewhere between the Foley bag of urine and a used bedpan. I found myself eye to eye with Mr. Wiszhinsky's pale, veined feet, which were buffeting about. Urine, stool, and foot odor; this, apparently, was where I ranked in the hospital hierarchy. Deservedly so, I had to agree. Even the nurse's aide knew how to drain the urine out of the Foley bag.

A foot massage! That's what I could do! Everybody likes a foot massage, and it might even be a way to help Mr. Wiszhinsky calm down. My childhood dog Kushi used to love it when I massaged her paws. She would smile her doggy smile and arch her back with pleasure as I rubbed two paws at a time. In any case, Mr. Wiszhinsky's feet were the only part I could get to; everybody else was focused on the action north of his belly button.

There was no one available to ask permission from. But, then again, there was no one to say I couldn't do it. There was no one, for that matter, to even notice my existence. Hoping I wouldn't cause too much trouble, I grabbed Mr. Wiszhinsky's feet. They were surprisingly smooth. I rubbed them gently at first to warm them up and then I started to massage them. I kneaded inside the arches and around the heels. I worked each toe separately. I rotated the ankles lightly. I thought I detected a trace of relaxation in his body.

I kept massaging while fluid crept out of his chest. The monitors stopped ringing and the warning lights stopped flashing. Mr. Wiszhinsky's limbs stopped flailing. His blood pressure came up and the decibel level of the crowd went down. The crisis was over.

Barely two hours on the medical service and I had witnessed a man nearly die, and then be saved. I walked out of Bellevue that night with my head swimming in a delirium of fluids and cardiogenic shock and pericardiocentesis. In front of the hulking brick hospital building was a small garden surrounded by a cast-iron fence. I walked along the meandering path lined with benches, thinking about that needle that had lanced through living, breathing skin. On the path was a graceful, multitiered fountain, now broken and filled with cigarette butts, and a birdbath resting on three legs carved of stone. The needle had punctured the borders of a human being, tearing through the boundaries of a life. In another circumstance it could be called assault, or attempted murder. But here, in this bizarre Bellevue world with remnants of Victorian elegance sitting side by side with glistening medical instruments, it was a workaday maneuver. The doctor hadn't even grimaced. I felt as though I had landed on a different planet.

⸎Mr. Wiszhinsky was transferred to the cardiac care unit (CCU). He improved dramatically after the fluid was removed from his heart, chatting with the nurses, watching TV, bickering with the orderlies. I doubted if he had even noticed that I'd been massaging his feet during the earlier commotion. I was just so happy that he was alive.

I spent a lot of time talking with Mr. and Mrs. Wiszhinsky—the familiarity of their Yiddish accents relaxed me. Mr. Wiszhinsky looked and spoke like my grandfather Irving, who had recently died of heart failure. Mr. Wiszhinsky told me about his life in Poland, life before the war. "Our town, she was so small," he said. "If you sneezed while walking on the road, you could miss it entirely. My father was the leatherman. Everything with leather. And our family worked in the shop, my mother, my sisters. We knew everything about leather. Even now I still remember. If you bring me the tools, I could make you a pair of shoes like you've never seen, in no time flat. What they have today in the stores they shouldn't even call shoes."

I told him about my grandfather's journey to America, his experience at Ellis Island. I told him how Irving and his brother sold fabric from a pushcart on the Lower East Side, bringing over their family from Latvia one by one. Eventually, they opened Reliable Silk, the fabric store in Mount Vernon that put my mother and her brothers through piano lessons, braces, and summer camp. We munched on the mandelbrot that Mrs. Wiszhinsky baked.

"*Oy*, and look at you now," he said, "a big doctor in a big fancy hospital. Your *zaydeh*, may he rest in peace, would be so proud. You should have this much *nachus* in your life always."

A unique bond is created, I learned, after you accompany someone through a lifesaving experience. Just by being near him and touching him during that near-death episode, I felt like I'd been privy to a singular intimacy. Mr. Wiszhinsky couldn't just recede into the multitudes of old men in the hospital, and I couldn't be just another medical student on the team. Not after we'd been so close to death together. Not after I'd touched his skin and felt the life racing through it while the needle bore into his heart, prying out the near-fatal fluid. And Mr. Wiszhinsky was special for another reason: he was my first patient on my first day at Bellevue. I'd walked through that teeming doorway into the world of Bellevue and Mr. Wiszhinsky was waiting for me, quivering on the margin of life and death. In an instant he'd drawn for me a stark demarcation line between being a scientist and being a physician. Our histories had collided and combined.

When my grandfather was dying of a failing heart, we had gathered with the doctor for the "family meeting." The doctor had said he'd have a few minutes at 8:00 in the morning so we got up early and assembled in the lounge. My grandmother, my mother, her two brothers—we sat in the vinyl upholstered chairs, drinking the free coffee that the hospital provided, making nervous jokes. Then the doctor came in, a young man, maybe in his thirties. Nobody spoke. My normally talkative family was silent. And so I asked how Irving was doing and the doctor directed his subsequent comments toward me. My family allowed me, without argument, to assume the role of medical emissary for them. But I was only a first-year medical student then, and my family couldn't have known how little I knew.

"He's in atrial fibrillation," the doctor said.

My family looked to me for a translation. I didn't want to disappoint them. "That means, uh ... that means the heart is fibrillating," I said, with extra emphasis on the last word so it would sound definitive. I recognized the term "fibrillation." I'd been in the medical environment long enough for "atrial fibrillation" to feel familiar on my tongue. I knew how to transpose the noun into a verb. But it was like a sentence gleaned from a foreign phrase book. I could memorize it, make it sound smooth and polished, but it wasn't truly absorbed into my own lexicon. Atrial fibrillation—I knew it was a term that I would soon understand, that would soon be part of my vernacular. That familiarity was so temptingly close. Too close to admit that I didn't actually know what fibrillation was, because I *almost* knew it. It was *almost* mine. The words were already physically comfortable in my mouth, but in reality I had no idea what atrial fibrillation was.

But I didn't want to disappoint. "That means the heart is fibrillating," was the best I could offer.

If only I could have fast-forwarded myself to the knowledge that I knew I was destined to acquire. Pericardial effusion—I knew the vocabulary word now as a third-year medical student. Cardiogenic shock—I tossed it off my tongue like I ordered my morning coffee in the coffee shop. But I still didn't really know what they meant.

∾I was concerned that I might be spending too much time chatting with Mr. Wiszhinsky about the old country and not enough time doing the real stuff that medical students do. Charlie and the other third-year students were busy fetching X-rays, shuttling stool samples to the lab, and drawing blood. I did, after all, want to get a good grade. I consulted my resident, Linda. She was a firm believer in the crucial role of the doctor-patient relationship in the healing process and encouraged my "nonmedical" activities with Mr. Wiszhinsky.

Linda told me that she had once taken care of an older Jewish man in the CCU. She and the patient had stayed up late every night talking. He'd told her stories about the old country and sang songs in Yiddish. I was relieved and heartened. So it was okay just to spend time with your patients. It was okay to do things beside record your patients' vital signs. My resident said so!

Mr. Wiszhinsky was in the CCU for almost a week. I spent most of my afternoons there shmoozing with him. One day, after a long conversation, he reached out and took my hand. I was touched and didn't pull back. He rolled toward me to give me a kiss on the cheek and I thought, "Well, this is okay, he's like my grandfather." Then he grabbed my chin and began kissing me on the lips. I tried to pull away but he held on tightly, kissing me harder and harder. His stale breath was hot on my skin as he pressed into me. He smelled like an old, sick man and the gray bristles of his unshaven beard scratched my cheek. I struggled to pull myself out, but I was tangled in his arms and the wires and the monitors.

The sour smell of sickness enveloped me and I crunched my eyes as tightly as I could to keep from vomiting. His fingers were digging into my jaw and his dry lips ground into mine. I clawed at him with my hands and twisted my body trying to disencumber myself. The wires caught in my hair and the blood pressure cuff on his arm snapped open. Finally I hurled my weight backward until I tumbled onto the floor and fled from the wretched CCU, fighting my way through the cardiology team that was just piling in for rounds and a dietary aide pushing a metal cart stacked with a tower of low-sodium lunch trays. A janitor was washing the hall in front of the CCU and he glared at me to stay away from the part he'd just cleaned. My stomach was coiling with nausea and I was desperate to get out. I took two steps forward but I was jostled through a sea of loud-talking residents who were squeezing through the narrow space allowed by the CAUTION— WET FLOOR signs. I could feel waves of sticky heat billowing up under my stiff white jacket. I just wanted to be someplace quiet and comforting. The doctors' station was filled with noisy interns debating the differential diagnosis of "palpable purpura." The nurses' station was crowded with medication carts and chart racks and clerks filing their nails. Phones were ringing and conversations were spinning and overhead announcements were blaring.

I finally sought refuge in the broom closet, the only quiet place I could find in this chaotic hospital. I slumped against the shelves of mops and sponges, panting in the dark. Disgust shivered through my body. I wanted to grab one of the cleansers off the shelf and wash him off me, his feeling, his smell, his breath.

How did everything get so twisted? I thought I'd been doing the right thing, spending quality time with my patient. Everybody was always telling us that doctors should spend more time with their patients. That's what all the good doctors did in books and the movies.

The walk home that night was lonely. Stretching up First Avenue was the collection of turn-of-the-century buildings that had all been part of Bellevue. They were grand, Gothic structures that could be elegant during the day, but at night—tonight—were eerie and forbidding. The imposing brick façades, with their nooks and crannies, balustrades and arches, loomed over me as I walked. The old psychiatric hospital was surrounded by a tall wrought-iron fence, and the walls were encased in dark velvet ivy. The building that was now the Bellevue men's shelter was set back behind a courtyard in disrepair. Four scalloped columns, like stranded emigrés from an ancient Greek temple, stuck out of the ground at various angles, forgotten by some renovation crew. Their flattened tops, supported by ornate and ominous curlicues, seemed preternaturally bare, as if begging for an offering or a sacrifice.

✑The next day before rounds I marched into the CCU. "Mr. Wiszhinsky," I said, trying to sound firm and controlled. "I am really angry. What you did to me yesterday wasn't right." I tightened my hands on my hips like a grade-school teacher chastising a tardy pupil. I paused righteously, waiting for his meek apology.

"It was your fault," he snapped, "you started it!"

I started it? Maybe letting him take my hand had been too suggestive. Maybe I'd worn something inappropriate yesterday. Maybe telling him about my family was something doctors weren't supposed to do. "I was just being nice to you."

"Eh, what nice?" he spat back. "You came in here. You started."

His week-old stubble and greasy, mussed hair rekindled shivers of loathing. "You are just a lecherous creep," I said. "You should be ashamed of yourself."

He shrugged, grumbled something in Yiddish, and then rolled toward the window. His motion caused static on the cardiac monitor and an alarm went off. I found myself staring at the liver spots on his back where the blue gown fell open. Two nurses rushed past me to fix the monitor. Beyond the bed, the window looked out over the East River. A gray angry sky tossed the water into jumbled waves. Pedestrians pulled themselves tighter into their coats to fight off the wind. Traffic was racing up the FDR Drive, oblivious to the cardiac monitors that were bleeping on the seventeenth floor of Bellevue. The hourly Circle Line Cruise filled with camera-toting tourists was heading north on the river. I had taken that cruise once before and I knew that the tour guide always pointed out Bellevue as one of the sites: "The oldest and craziest hospital in the nation." I sighed and walked out of the CCU.

I didn't see Mr. Wiszhinsky much after that, except briefly on morning rounds. If I had to speak to him I tried my best to sound cool and professional. He looked so pathetic in his hospital-issue pajamas and green Styrofoam slippers that it was hard to stay mad. Stuck in that bed, strapped in by endless wires and monitors, stripped of his usual surroundings and his own clothing, eating bland food without an iota of sodium or cholesterol, listening to nurses and doctors who were probably one-third his age talk to him with condescending cheeriness. Were his actions the only way he could rebel against the indignities of being sick?

I had pangs of longing for my research laboratory where I'd spent years amid the familiarity and security of the scientific paraphernalia. There was something reassuring about the crisp friction of clean glass test tubes in my hand, waiting for a new experiment to begin. The buffer solutions that I prepared contained fixed ingredients in reliable proportions. The chemical structures of the compounds I used were steady and dependable; I could count on them. Not so, it seemed, with patients. Passing through that narrow, crowded doorway of Bellevue had pitched me into a world that was heady and tremulous. I couldn't control the parameters as I did during my experiments in the lab. There I could hold all conditions constant and vary only the one I wished to study. Entering Bellevue was like being in a lab experiment gone wild, with every possible parameter running amok. Knowledge would not be coming in an orderly, logical progression. But during that first chaotic week of medicine I conquered that most harrowing medical student hurdle: I learned how to draw blood. And Zalman Wiszhinsky was my first victim.

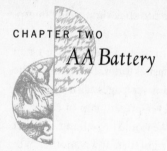

CHAPTER TWO

AA Battery

"Nine P.M.," somebody shouted. "Rikers bus rollin' in!"

I stepped out of the Bellevue ER into the chilly spring night to see what the excitement was. Just pulling in was a school bus, the kind I'd taken every day in elementary school, but this one was light blue instead of yellow. Boxy letters stenciled in midnight blue draped over the metallic ridges that ran along the sides of the bus: NEW YORK CITY DEPARTMENT OF CORRECTIONS. All the windows and doors were covered with double layers of thick metal mesh. Squinting, I could make out vague silhouettes of heads and shoulders inside. It was a cage on wheels.

Twelve young men bound in hand- and legcuffs sauntered out. They were connected by a twenty-foot metal chain that threaded through each of their shackles. The long chain dragged and clattered against the ground as they walked—the twelve of them joined as one unwieldy, serpentine organism. A few threw back their shoulders and jutted their hips forward in an attempted swagger, but their steps were snapped back by the chains. I was the only other person standing outside other than the correctional officers. Each prisoner seemed to eye me specifically and deliberately as he walked by. I shuddered and hurried inside, glad to have the freedom to rejoin the noise and chaos of the ER.

It was my very first night on call. Even the words impressed me: "on call." Now I, too, could comment casually about my morning fatigue: "Oh, I was 'on call' last night." I wasn't actually sure what I was supposed to do while on call, but I knew I had to stick tight to my intern, Li-Chan.

I soon learned that following an intern was no easy task. Li-Chan walked, breathed, and existed twice as fast as I did. She could write notes on her scut list with one hand, answer pages with the other, eat a bagel, and somehow not spill her ever-present cup of coffee. At times her movements were a blur to me. We would be walking together and she would suddenly execute a sharp right turn down another hallway. It would be several steps before I realized that I was now walking alone. My life seemed to consist of racing to catch up with her.

Li-Chan had a petite build, but when she strode down the corridor with the tails of her white coat whipping behind her, patients, nurses, and visitors shrank out of her way. Her white coat had that blasé worn look that I so envied. The smudges and wrinkles and stains bespoke weighty duties that surmounted any possible fashion statement a crisp clean coat could offer. Li-Chan wore the sleeves crammed up past her elbows, ready for important intern work at a moment's notice.

The coat itself was a monument to economy and proficiency. The side pockets bulged with syringes, gauze pads, alcohol swabs, and IVs. The breast pocket was jammed with index cards, pens, EKG calipers, and the tiny blue *Facts and Formulas* book. The eighty-two pages of microscopic print in that three-by-five-inch book contained everything from disorders of phosphorous metabolism to the calculations for fractional excretion of sodium. Page 30 was folded over for rapid access to Renal Tubular Acidosis—every intern had to be able to distinguish Type IV RTA from Types I and II. There never seemed to be any discussion of Type III.

Li-Chan's beeper was clipped to the outside of that same breast pocket so that the numbers on the tiny screen would be within reading distance and at the appropriate orientation for instant response. In addition to the regular pockets of the white coat, there were side-slit pockets that allowed access to one's pants pockets. Clamped onto Li-Chan's left side-slit was a needle-nosed metal hemostat that secured a roll of cloth tape. It reminded me of the way we used to carry toilet paper on overnight hikes in summer camp.

No intern, of course, would ever be caught dead with a buttoned-up coat; that was only for attending physicians who were too idle to actually require the immediate proximity of equipment in their pockets. And so even the buttonholes of Li-Chan's white coat were corralled into use. A reflex hammer with a red rubber nose dangled through the topmost buttonhole. A rubber tourniquet for drawing blood was tied through the second. And a large silver barrette was pinned through the last. When the duty of clinical medicine called, Li-Chan would whip out that barrette and crisply snap her long hair out of the way. As soon as she was finished inserting an IV or saving someone's life, that barrette would be clipped back into its proper place until the next procedure.

Li-Chan's efficiency extended to her speech as well. She only spoke when it was necessary, and then only with the precise pithy words that were needed. She and our resident, Linda, could review the entire medical situation of their patient with just a few terse phrases. "Rivera—get another set of numbers, repeat films . . . Carson—call GI, get her scoped . . . Santos—M11Q for dispo, turf to geriatrics." Li-Chan would march off to accomplish these tasks and I'd scramble along after her like I was supposed to. I wanted to know what was going on, but I knew she had important things to do and I didn't want to slow her down with questions. I couldn't tell if Li-Chan disliked me or was just too busy to notice my presence.

"A spring intern," Linda smiled when I expressed my difficulty keeping up with Li-Chan. "There's nothing like a solid spring intern." I hung my head, my seasons woefully out of sync. I wasn't a spring medical student at all. March was nearly ending and the cherry trees in front of NYU were just starting to bud, but I still didn't know how to get stat X-rays done or where to find the cardiology fellows when they wouldn't answer their pages. I was really a July greenhorn student. I had only just learned how to draw blood on Mr. Wiszhinsky. And it still took me two or three sticks.

I wanted desperately to be a useful member of the team, but I had nothing to contribute to the rapid-fire efficiency of patient care at Bellevue. Whenever I asked to help I always noticed a slight hesitation in Li-Chan's reply. That micro-second of a pause reinforced just how much of a burden I was, how much of an impediment I was to the functioning of the well-oiled medical machine. Her eyes would briefly flit away from my gaze and I could tell that she was debating whether the possible gain from my assistance would be worth the time lost in explaining to me what to do. I felt guilty asking to help, but I felt guilty standing around watching Li-Chan juggle six tasks at once. I felt guilty just existing.

∽Linda announced that we had an admission. An admission! A real patient! We would take a history, do a physical exam, interpret the diagnostic tests, then write a beautifully detailed admission note in the chart. Li-Chan rolled her eyes and tugged another sheet of paper from her overstuffed clipboard. Being the solid spring intern that she was, Li-Chan didn't require Linda's oversight for the admission so she and I were sent off alone. "On autopilot," Linda had said to me with a shrug. Linda disappeared to handle more weighty matters in the CCU.

Li-Chan spit out her chewing gum into a 4x4 gauze pad that she'd fished from one of her pockets. "It's a Rikers guy," she said. "Says here on the transfer note that he swallowed an AA battery and a wood screw."

"An AA battery and a wood screw?" I asked. "Why would anyone do that?"

Li-Chan reached into another pocket and extracted three sugar packets. She grasped them together and nicked them open with her teeth. Inverting them, she carefully aimed the stream of sugar into the hole that she'd torn in the plastic cover of her coffee cup. "To get out of jail. They all do it." A tongue depressor emerged from her breast pocket. She jammed the wooden blade through the hole and stirred in the sugar. "Half the time they're lying anyway, but Rikers has to send them over for evaluation no matter what." Li-Chan tipped her head back and guzzled some coffee. "It's called a Bellevue vacation."

Balancing her coffee cup and clipboard in her left hand, Li-Chan smoothly eased an X-ray out of its gangly paper folder with her right hand and popped it onto the lightbox. I had never read a chest X-ray before, but even I couldn't miss this one. There, in the upper left-hand corner of the stomach area, was a clearly outlined AA battery. And in the upper right hand corner was a two-inch screw. I could even see the threads.

Ben Harwood was sitting sullenly on a gurney in the corner of the ER. His torso was hunched over manacled wrists. His baby-blue hospital gown had slipped open at the back, revealing iridescent brown skin. The muscles of his back were sleekly accentuated, and they glistened with the light each time he shifted his body. He was well over six feet tall, but he had rounded himself over into a small, compact ball. His hair was cropped close to his scalp and his eyes were shadowed by a heavy brow. He stared down at the floor. The two burly, white officers guarding him were sharing a bag of potato chips. All three turned to watch us as we approached: two women, each under 120 pounds, sporting white coats and stethoscopes.

One of the officers hitched his pants up over his paunch and narrowed his eyes. "You the doctors?" Li-Chan plunked her coffee cup on the nightstand and nodded firmly. I stared down at the foot of the IV pole. The officer looked at his partner for a moment and then turned back at us. "This here Harwood says he swallowed some stuff. What's the verdict?"

Li-Chan turned to the prisoner. "The X-ray shows a battery in your stomach and a screw in your intestine. Why did you swallow them?"

Mr. Harwood looked back down at the floor. "Dunno. Just felt like it, I guess."

The second officer butted in. "Don't listen to him. He just wanted to get out of the can for a while."

Li-Chan ignored the officer. "Were you trying to kill yourself?"

"I dunno." Mr. Harwood continued to stare downward. "Nah, just bein' stupid, I guess."

"How old are you, Mr. Harwood?" I asked.

"Seventeen."

"Just made the cut-off for Rikers," chimed in the first officer, tilting back the bag of chips so that the last few crumbs trickled into his mouth.

"We'll take our own history, thank you very much," Li-Chan snapped at the officer. She turned back to Mr. Harwood. "Ever been sick before? Diabetes? Asthma? Hepatitis?" The patient didn't react and Li-Chan seemed to take that as a "no" to her questions. "Any surgeries? Take any meds? Got any allergies to meds? Anything run in your family? Do you smoke, drink, or take drugs?" I couldn't tell if Mr. Harwood was even registering her questions, but it was the fastest history I'd yet seen. "All right," Li-Chan said, "we're going to draw some blood and do some tests." With that, she spun on her heel and marched off to the supply room. It took me a moment to realize that she was already gone and I sprang up to follow her.

✑Mr. Harwood and the two officers settled into a back corner of the ER. The old ER was a maze of dreary rooms on the ground floor of the hospital. At the back were the sliding glass doors where the ambulances pulled up to drop off their victims. The triage area was the adjacent hallway where the stretchers accumulated. The nurses made their way down the queue assessing the patients, pulling forward those with chest pain and shortness of breath and leaving those with stomachaches to wait it out. The line itself was a mirror of New York City. There were white business executives with heart attacks, tattooed heroin addicts sleeping off their hits, European tourists with Gucci bags and food poisoning, suburban teenagers who'd done uppers or downers or both at Greenwich Village bars that didn't check ID, African and Asian immigrants with strange parasitic infections, AIDS patients with roaring fevers, old ladies hit by taxi cabs while crossing the street, off-the-boat Central Americans with rare diseases who came to the United States with the name "Bellevue" scrawled on a piece of paper, pregnant teenagers with no prenatal care having their first contractions, middle-aged Bangladeshis with craggy cholesterol-laden coronary arteries, Black teenagers with asthma attacks, Tibetan monks who'd been on hunger strikes in front of the nearby United Nations, and the alcoholics who reeked of Thunderbird and knew all the nurses by their first names.

The line of stretchers led into the tiny windowless corner where the doctors evaluated the patients. Eight stretchers could squeeze in at a time, each separated by a three-quarter length curtain. Often the patients would be surrounded by whole teams of residents, interns, and students who found themselves jostling hips and backs with other teams of residents, interns, and students on the other side of the curtain evaluating their own patient. Through the bottoms of the curtains, scrub-clad legs and surgical clogs peered out, mixing with spilled gauze pads, brown stains of iodine, and the blue plastic bags holding patients' possessions that were tucked under each of the stretchers.

There was no decrement of voice from one "room" to the next so adjacent conversations and medical histories blended easily. "*Dolor?* Do you have any *dolor, señor?*" "Anybody speak Cantonese?" "How much insulin do you take?"

Bits of sound drifted freely under the curtains: the rubber slurp of EKG bulbs sucking onto a chest, the snap of latex gloves, the clink of blood tubes. And the smells of rubbing alcohol, drinking alcohol, and homelessness filtered easily about the small space. Toxic sock syndrome, the interns liked to joke.

Patients who were stable and just waiting for beds upstairs languished in the SOU—the Satellite Observation Unit—which was really the same open hallway as Triage. Patients who were clinically unstable were wheeled through a narrow door to the EW—the Emergency Ward—a section that was equipped like an intensive care unit but far more cramped and dank than the real ICU upstairs. There were no windows and the walls were painted a grubby, depressing shade of green. A single white counter, sticky from generations of spilled coffee, was the only work space for nurses, doctors, and students alike.

A small corner of the Triage area was reserved for asthmatics to receive their nebulizers. Nearby was a procedure room to do suturing, spinal taps, and central venous lines.

In the middle of the ER was the trauma slot, set aside for the disasters. "Slot" was the noun that represented both the actual room ("He's in the slot") or the patient ("There's a slot coming in"). It was also the verb ("They slotted Mr. Hanson"). Everyone in the ER knew when a slot was coming in. Actually, everyone in the entire hospital knew when a slot was coming in because the page operators would make particularly well-articulated overhead announcements when paging the appropriate team of doctors to the slot phone extension: 4344. No one ever actually had to call the number, they just dashed straight to the slot upon hearing it announced. The fun was guessing what the slot was by who was paged. "Trauma, orthopedics, 4344 stat" was usually a car accident. "Trauma, neurosurgery, 4344 stat" was either a gunshot to the head or a head-on collision. "Medical consult, 4344 stat" was a cardiac arrest. "Trauma, OB-GYN, 4344 stat" was anything that happened to a pregnant woman.

One time there was a man who had jumped out of a four-story window. I tried to peek into the mass, but as usual, I saw only jostling, scrub-clad, backs. A paramedic was standing nearby and saw my craning neck. "This guy never would've made it," he said, jerking his head toward the patient who was swamped with doctors, "if it wasn't for them good New York City mice." He pointed his finger toward a gray smudge on the floor. "Landed on a mouse, this guy. Landed on a mouse and slid like he was on ice instead of being smashed to smithereens." He pursed his lips and nodded thoughtfully. "Saved his life, but I can't say the same for the mouse." I looked closer at the gray smudge. It was a flattened, bloody mat of fur. A mouse that had probably started its life in the wilds of Central Park, strayed onto the sidewalks, ended up under someone's suicidal shoe, and then traveled by ambulance to end its days in the Bellevue trauma slot.

The ER was big and crowded, but small when it came to gossip. Word spread quickly about the battery and the wood screw—everyone seemed to be in the know. Nurses and clerks were chatting about it. I overheard an intern joke about loose screws. Some big GI attending was coming in all the way from his home to fish out the battery and the screw with an endoscope. Li-Chan wheeled Mr. Harwood to the EW, since endoscopy was considered "serious stuff" that might require more "serious" monitoring.

This was going to be exciting.

The GI attending was a short, balding man with a nasal voice. His head sunk straight into his shoulders without benefit of much neck. His belly spilled generously over his belt, obscuring his beeper and waistline. Next to Mr. Harwood's sleek, muscled body, he looked like a troll from a fairy tale. The GI attending scanned the room and saw me standing there, hands in my pockets. "You," he said, "get some saline. Make it fast." Saline? Where's saline? Panicked, I flagged down the nearest nurse's aide and asked for saline. She handed me a slurpy plastic IV bag that I quickly deposited in front of the attending.

He snorted. "Not IV saline; I'm not running an IV department over here." He craned his pudgy neck and looked about the room with a wider angle. "Can somebody please get me a bottle of sterile saline so I can start this procedure already?" Li-Chan strode behind the nurses' desk without even asking the nurse for permission and snagged a plastic liter bottle out of the glass cabinet. She opened the top with a sharp crack and plopped it on the endoscopy cart. A spring intern. I edged further away from the attending, hoping to be camouflaged by the cardiac monitors—a July medical student mistakenly deposited into March.

The attending rolled up his sleeves. He slung his arms through a baby-blue patient gown to protect his shirt and tie so that Mr. Harwood and the GI attending were now wearing matching outfits.

The attending waved the endoscope in front of Mr. Harwood. It was a three-foot tube, about one-half inch in diameter, with a fiberoptic camera inside. "See this, young man? We are going to insert this through your mouth and down into your stomach to pull those things out. The most important thing is not to bite down on the scope as it goes in. Do you hear me? Don't bite on the scope." Mr. Harwood grunted what I supposed was an assent.

Li-Chan injected a sedative into Mr. Harwood's IV. After a few minutes, his eyes drooped and he slumped back on the stretcher. The GI attending knuckled him once on the chest, and when he got no response began threading the huge endoscope into Mr. Harwood's mouth.

As the endoscope entered his mouth Mr. Harwood's eyes flew open and his teeth clamped down on the tube, despite the plastic protective mouthpiece he'd been given. He bolted upward, grabbing at the endoscope.

The GI attending jumped back and yelled, "This is a ten thousand dollar instrument, young man. Get your hands off of it." Struggling to get the scope out of Mr. Harwood's grip he snapped at Li-Chan and me, "Sedate this man, will you?"

Li-Chan whipped another syringe out of her pocket and injected a stronger sedative. We waited until Mr. Harwood was clearly drowsy. He answered our questions in a slurred voice and his head lolled backward. As soon as the GI attending inserted the endoscope, however, Mr. Harwood shook his bulk and fought his way through the sedative to grab at the tube.

"Nurse!" cried the attending. "I need full restraints here." Two to a limb, four nurses tied each of Mr. Harwood's trunk-like arms to the bed. Li-Chan injected another sedative. After ten minutes, Mr. Harwood was asleep. He didn't respond to any of Li-Chan's pokes and prods with a needle.

The GI attending pushed up his sleeves and began to snake the endoscope in once again. Mr. Harwood shuddered violently and strained his manacled limbs. Saliva spilled down his cheeks as he gnashed at the endoscope. The GI attending persevered, pressing the tube into the patient's mouth. The attending's thinning hair, which had been carefully combed over the balding scalp, fell forward in sticky strands onto his sweaty forehead. Mr. Harwood continued to buck.

"Get this guy down," the attending snarled. "I don't care what it takes. Just keep him from biting my scope."

"He's probably a heavy drug user." Li-Chan shrugged. "He's tolerant to all these sedatives."

"Whatever," grumbled the GI attending, "just knock him out."

"He'll be at risk for respiratory suppression with all these drugs. He could aspirate all that saliva into his lungs."

"Then call anesthesia," the attending barked at Li-Chan. "Paralyze him! Intubate him if you have to! I don't care. I just want to get my job done without my equipment being destroyed." The attending's gown hadn't been fastened properly and was beginning to loosen and slip down his arms. As he moved about, the baby-blue gown with the delicate floral pattern bunched over his belly. The folds of polyester piled up, threatening to slide over his abdominal precipice at any moment.

The anesthesia resident arrived promptly with a large metal toolbox. A blue cap was pulled tight over his head and a crumpled surgical mask dangled from his neck. Muttering to himself, he whisked out several fierce-looking syringes and discharged them promptly into the IV. I watched Mr. Harwood's body shiver, then slowly melt into silence. His head sank back against the pillow and his eyelids, which had been tightly scrunched shut, now lay softly closed. The resident held Mr. Harwood's chin open with his left hand and unsnapped a stiff metal lever with his right. He slipped the lever in and jerked up Mr. Harwood's jaw with such force that I thought teeth would fly out. The resident leaned in and peered deep into the mouth—he and Mr. Harwood were nose to nose. Without diverting his gaze, the resident grabbed for a long plastic tube from his toolbox and jammed it down the throat. He took a quick listen to Mr. Harwood's lungs with his stethoscope to make sure the breathing tube was in place, then he sat back and stretched his neck with a satisfying crack. He snapped the metal lever shut. "All yours," he said, and strode away with his toolbox in tow.

Between the breathing machine, the endoscopy cart, the cardiac monitor, the GI attending, and Li-Chan, there was barely room for me to squeeze in. The two police officers sat at the foot of the bed reading the *New York Post*.

The attending managed to thread the endoscope through Mr. Harwood's mouth and into his stomach, and suddenly a color picture flashed up on the attached video monitor. The inside of the stomach was lined with glistening pink ridges. Liquid swished about, intermittently blurring the view. A greenish thing floated by. "Must've had lettuce for dinner," Li-Chan said. The camera careened around the stomach. I was getting queasy.

Then a black cylinder popped into view. "There it is," cried out the

GI attending. I squeezed in closer to get a look at the screen. "Pana-sonic AA" glittered on the side of the battery.

A metal claw appeared on the screen, reaching out from the endo-scope. The images lurched about as the claw chased the battery in Mr. Harwood's stomach. The attending sucked in his cheeks as he maneu-vered the controls on the endoscope. Mr. Harwood had started to fid-get but the attending didn't notice; his eyes were glued to the screen. He pursued the battery around the curves of the stomach, swishing his way through Rikers cuisine, his baby-blue gown teetering over the edge.

Suddenly, the GI attending let out a hoot of victory—the claw had nabbed its prey. The black snake rapidly retreated with the Panasonic battery in its fangs. On the screen the images of Mr. Harwood's stom-ach and esophagus reeled backward in dizzying succession. The endo-scope slithered its way out through Mr. Harwood's mouth and all at once the battery appeared in real life, dangling in the air. The claw re-leased its grip and the battery was plunked triumphantly into a plastic urine specimen cup. The attending smiled and rested his elbows on the endoscopy machine.

The screw was apparently too far along to be reached. It would have to pass of its own accord. "Just run your hands through each of his bowel movements," the GI attending cheerily called out to us as he wheeled the endoscopy cart out of the ER, his gown sagging nearly to his knees.

Li-Chan and I were left alone with Mr. Harwood. Despite the breathing tube, the handcuffs, the cloth restraints, and the untold number of sedatives, he still squirmed in the bed. He drooled thick sputum as he mumbled incoherently.

Li-Chan turned to me. "Okay, he needs an arterial blood gas. You want to do it?"

Me? A blood gas? I would actually do something for a patient?

I fumbled with the syringe, trying to get the butterfly needle hooked up without pricking myself but it accidentally flopped against the bed-sheets, rendering it unsterile. I fished in my pocket for another butterfly needle package, but it was the wrong size. Li-Chan pulled one out of her pocket and wordlessly handed it to me. Mr. Harwood was contorting on the bed. I held the needle and syringe in one hand with the needle pointed upward so it would stay sterile, then tried to open the gauze pads with the other hand. But I had no free fingers, so I reached with my teeth. Li-Chan snapped the gauze pads out of my hand and tore them open for me. I peered at the cloth restraints; they seemed a bit rickety against Mr. Harwood's straining wrists. I had never drawn blood from an artery before. Veins were relatively easy to draw blood from because they sat on the surface and could actually be visualized. Arteries, on the other hand, lay much deeper in the tissue. They could only be identified by feeling for the pulse, then one had to plunge the needle straight down into the wrist, deep into the layers of muscle and tendon, relying as much on intuition as on faith. Arteries also could bleed much more ferociously than veins, since the pressure of the heart beating would continually force blood out of the wound unless compressed hard and long.

"You know . . ." I started. Mr. Harwood ground his teeth against the breathing tube. I reached for an alcohol swab and accidentally knocked the gauze pads to the floor. "Maybe this isn't the best patient to learn on." Mr. Harwood's torso arched upward and I could see his shoulder muscles bulging. "Maybe I'll watch you do it this time and then try it next time." I bent over to grab for the fallen gauze pads and my white coat swept against the butterfly needle. Unsterile again.

"Whatever . . ." Li-Chan unwrapped a piece of chewing gum. "You forgot the heparin anyway—the blood would've clotted." She broke open a new syringe and filled it with heparin. In three seconds she had the butterfly opened and hooked up to the syringe, the alcohol swabs and gauze pads neatly lined up, and a strip of surgical tape hanging from the table to secure the bandage at the end of the procedure. "Just help me hold his arm still."

Li-Chan and I grabbed hold of Mr. Harwood's twisting left arm and tried to immobilize it in the proper position—flat, open forearm with the palm bent all the way back to expose the wrist. Mr. Harwood reared into the air, pulling the sheets with him. He dislodged his arm from our grip with a violent shake. Li-Chan tried to push him back onto the bed while I struggled to grasp the writhing arm.

"Do you think you guys could give us a hand over here?" Li-Chan called out to the two police officers who were engrossed in the cross-word puzzle.

They pulled themselves up quickly, looking a bit sheepish. "Sorry ma'am. We're not allowed to interfere with the prisoner's medical treatment."

Mr. Harwood continued to buck. "I think we are finished with the medical treatment," Li-Chan said. "Now we're just having some friendly wrestling."

The officers looked down and stammered something unintelligible. Two ER nurses came to our assistance and pinned Mr. Harwood down. Li-Chan touched one finger near the pulse in his wrist and sank the needle deep into his wrist without even a pause. Bright red arterial blood pulsed immediately into the plastic tubing of the butterfly. Before I could even take note of her technique, the needle was out and the bandage securely taped on. Li-Chan gave me his wrist to hold while she fetched ice for the blood sample. "Press for five minutes. Don't let up, not even for one second."

I grasped Mr. Harwood's hand in mine, pressing as hard as I could on his wrist. He groaned a few more times, then finally fell asleep, utterly exhausted. The nurses scurried around him, checking his blood pressure, pulse, and temperature, suctioning out his breathing tube. The plastic urine cup sat upon the ventilator, calmly displaying the AA battery.

After the breathing tube was removed, Mr. Harwood was transferred upstairs to 16-North. He was placed in a four-bedded room, but there were no roommates. One of his legs was always cuffed to the bed by a few inches of chain. The urinal and bedpan were parked within arm's reach. A police guard sat outside the room twenty-four hours a day, sleeping or reading the *New York Post*.

Mostly Mr. Harwood sat hunched on the edge of the bed, facing away from the row of windows that offered spectacular views of the East River. I tried several times to engage him in conversation, but to my questions he only grunted monosyllabically. He intimated that he had been in psychiatric hospitals before. He mentioned that he'd tried to hang himself. Then slashed his wrists. "Once ate a few thumbtacks," he mumbled.

He sat in the same position for the three days of his stay on the medical ward, his forearms resting on his thighs, his head hanging toward the ground. A stretch of his neck lay exposed in that position and there was something so tender about it, so vulnerable. Such a powerful body, weighted down into a snail-shell, chained to the railing, with just that bit of neck exposed to the world. I stood next to him, after yet another series of unanswered questions, looking at that sliver of neck. Could I just place my hand there? What would it feel like? My fingertips hovered in the air. With Mr. Wiszhinsky it had been easier; he had been writhing in pain when the fluid was drawn from his heart and seemed to be calling out for some human touch. But Ben Harwood was so curled into himself, so folded into his space, that I couldn't bring myself to intrude. It seemed that he had carved out a solitary spot, fortified it with the muscles of his body, and created a protected shelter for his soul. I pulled my hand back. It wasn't my place to breech those defended borders.

∞Each morning on rounds we examined Mr. Harwood's daily abdominal X-ray. We watched the two-inch wood screw wend its way down his intestines. On the third day it was gone. We never caught it in the bedpan.

After the wood screw had passed and it was clear that he was in no further medical danger, he was transferred to the psychiatry ward. I never saw him again.

I wondered if Mr. Harwood would talk to the psychiatrists. I envisioned him sitting exactly the same way as he'd been on the medical ward, like a tortoise in his shell. The psychiatrists would talk at him, around him. Maybe medicate him. I wondered if he would ever share his history and allow himself to get help. How long could a person live with that inside them? Even a person with ramparts as strong as the Greek columns outside of Bellevue.

His battery, in its plastic urine cup, had been brought to our doctor's station to show our attending on rounds. Then it sat there, occasionally the butt of an intern's joke when someone's beeper needed a new battery. Then it was forgotten, absorbed into the general mess of the doctors' station—stray X-rays, crumpled progress notes, unused blood tubes. A few weeks later I returned to that doctors' station; somebody had cleaned up. The blood tubes and IVs were collected in plastic bins and sorted by size. The books and manuals were lined up neatly on the shelf. And the battery in its urine cup was gone.

CHAPTER THREE

Stuck

My tears must stop, for every drop
Hinders needle and thread.

Thomas Hood, "The Song of the Shirt"

"HEY, WAKE UP," a voice barked, as my shoulder was shaken roughly. Weighted in a warm thick sleep, my body refused to acknowledge the outside world

The shaking continued. "Get up, we've got a case."

I rolled away from the intrusions, sinking back toward the heavy swamplike inertia of sleep. The density of my body submerged lower and lower, away from the chilly outside.

"Listen, I don't have time for this." The shaking of my shoulder intensified and now rattled through to my torso. "A case is starting and you've got to be there."

"What?" I mumbled, pulling the paper gown that was my blanket higher up on my body. It crinkled and slipped, allowing some of the precious, sleepy warmth to seep out.

"Come on, get up. There's a hysterectomy on the table and the attending said to get the medical students." With a slow throb my eyes opened. In the dim light I could just barely make out one of the OB-GYN interns. Was it Sam? Or Michael? I could barely keep track of who was who when I was fully awake, let alone asleep. "Come on," he repeated, "they're already prepping her. I gotta run and get scrubbed." Probably Sam—the one who was always itching to get into the OR.

"Okay," I grumbled. "I'll be there." I shivered, trying to adjust my eyes to the room. The OB-GYN call room was windowless. The lightbulbs couldn't have generated more than twenty watts. There was one bed for the intern. It had a mattress that sagged low in the middle. But I longed for that saggy bed, since the students only merited mattresses that were strewn haphazardly on the floor. For the first few nights I was too afraid to sleep, convinced that there were rats lurking in the perpetually dim room. But by the end of the first week I was too tired to keep vigil.

Sheets were a challenge. I think the nurses deliberately hid them from the medical students. And blankets—there wasn't even a chance. During the day it wasn't a problem, but as soon as night fell and all the regular employees went home, the temperature began its insidious descent. As the hospital emptied out, leaving only the housestaff, students, and nightshift staff, it grew steadily colder. Some people said that the cold feeling was just from being tired, but I was convinced that there was a more organized conspiracy at work. Somewhere in the bowels of Bellevue resided the Chief of Arctic Controls. He sat perched on a wooden stool and stared at his watch. As each hour passed he would click the thermostat down another notch. With a flourish, I was sure. Down and down that thermostat would go until I would awaken at three in the morning to find the tips of my fingers blue with numbness.

I wore a T-shirt under my cloth scrubs. And paper scrubs over the cloth scrubs. And a sweatshirt on top of the paper scrubs. My white jacket was on top of everything and still I was cold. In desperation I'd snagged a sterile surgical gown from the supply closet to cover myself. The gowns were made of paper, but they were thick and I was able to wrap the extra-large size twice around my body. I'm sure that using sterile gowns as blankets would not be considered a cost-effective use of resources by the Bellevue administration, but I was just too damn cold to care.

My hand ventured out from under the paper gown and fished around on the chilly linoleum for my glasses. I had long since given up wearing contact lenses on the OB-GYN rotation since I had to sleep overnight in the hospital so often. And of course there was the issue of protecting my eyes from blood and body fluids—the delivery rooms and OR were notorious for reckless fluids. I located my glasses and eased them onto my face. They had chilled sitting on the floor and the icy metal frames stung.

I staggered out from the call room into the brightly lit hallway, blinking and shivering. I had no idea what time it was—only that it was some time between midnight and sunrise. I waded through my grogginess down the empty hallway toward the OR.

What was I doing here, on this ward, in the middle of the night, in subzero weather? That's right, OB-GYN. Medical student. On call. Hysterectomy.

I'd only been on this rotation for three weeks but any enthusiasm I'd started with had already been wrung out of my body. OB-GYN wasn't anything like my medicine rotation. On medicine I was part of a team and followed Li-Chan for the entire time. I was always on call with Li-Chan, even if she didn't always acknowledge my presence. I had regular patients whom I rounded on every day. I took their blood pressure and listened to their lungs each morning. I wrote daily progress notes in their charts. Every day the attendings met with us to review our cases. At noon there was always an academic conference. The work was overwhelming, but the people and the schedule were consistent. Once I got the hang of the system, I had something to rely on for the twelve weeks.

OB-GYN was like chasing spilled mercury from a thermometer. For my entire eight weeks I struggled with the slippery chaotic elements. I never knew where I was supposed to be, who I was supposed to be following, what exactly were my responsibilities. Unlike medicine, I wasn't assigned to any particular human being. On one day I'd follow Michael, then he'd get busy with a complicated labor case and patch me off to Sam, the other intern. He'd let me trot after him until there was a good case in the OR and he'd disappear. Then I'd find Ellen, the second-year resident. But she'd be too tired from her night on call and she'd send me over to Warren, the chief resident. Warren would give me a halfhearted lecture on placenta biology, but then he'd have to attend some administrative meeting and he'd tell me to go find a midwife to follow around. The midwives, however, were particularly concerned about providing their patients with a holistic and soothing environment. Medical students were considered neither holistic nor soothing and I was generally ignored until I eventually wandered elsewhere.

I felt like I was constantly stretching and twisting, contorting to gather the escaping fragments into a recognizable and understandable order. But I could never grasp one part without another slithering from my grip.

There was the unpredictable disorganization of the obstetrics section—endless hours drawing blood, placing IVs, ferrying samples down to the lab. Then somebody would holler "Delivery!" or "C-section!" Suddenly the intern would come flying down the hall, tossing off his white coat as he ran. The nurses would scramble into the patient's room to arrange the monitoring devices and prepare to transfer the patient. The chief resident would yell orders at the nurses. The stretchers of the overflow patients who had been parked in the hallway would be clanked and jolted into a new formation to allow the gathering tempest to escape. Before I could figure out what was happening, a stretcher with a howling woman perched atop would barrel down the hall surrounded by a mass of sprinting figures in blue scrubs all hanging on to the rails. I'd rush over to catch the moving train. But I was never sure where to place my body. Behind the intern? Next to the chief resident? In front of the nurse? Next to the IV pole? Half the time the baby was already out before I'd even finished scrubbing.

Chasing slippery balls of mercury.

Then there was the gynecology section, which was mainly long, grueling hours watching surgery in the OR. Every fourth night I slept on a mattress on the floor of that freezing, grimy, windowless room. I didn't dare contemplate how old those mattresses were or what creatures might live inside. Sleep wasn't actually what happened, since the interns constantly dragged me out of bed to draw blood. Drawing blood seemed to be the *raison d'être* of the medical students. Luckily, pregnant patients were known for their plump, juicy veins and they were "easy sticks"—nothing like the first time I'd tried to draw blood from Mr. Wiszhinsky. By the middle of the rotation I was a pro.

The OB-GYN patients themselves were a blur to me. In and out of the ward they would slide. I'd draw their blood and then they'd be gone before I'd even learned their names. I'd place an IV and when I'd gotten back from lunch their surgery would already have been finished or their baby already delivered. I was rarely able to actually follow a patient from beginning to end as I'd done with Zalman Wiszhinsky and Ben Harwood. Patients floated in and out, residents disappeared and reappeared—there was no chance for people to click and hold, no chance for lives to engage long enough to make indelible marks. Only, it seemed, a never-ending struggle with fatigue and cold.

From the anteroom where the scrub sinks were, I could see a woman being wheeled in on a gurney. She was surrounded by nurses and doctors all clad in scrubs, masks, and gowns. Although I was only a few feet away, it was impossible to recognize anybody in the mass of blue coverings.

I dreaded shedding my excess clothing and losing the few particles of warmth that I'd struggled to accumulate. I peeled off my white coat and then my sweatshirt, the chill of my fatigue penetrating deeper with each layer I removed. Gingerly I removed the oversized paper scrubs until I was left in just a short-sleeve top. Moving more quickly now to shake off the cold, I crammed my hair up into one of those ridiculous shower caps and pulled paper booties over my sneakers. My fingers fumbled with the slippery strings trying to tie the mask over my mouth and nose. Finally I kicked on the faucet with the foot lever.

Hot water.

I took in a long delicious breath. The water rippled over my arms, smoothing off the goose pimples. The blue of my fingers gave way to pink and then to red. My skin unfurled its pores toward the geyser of steaming water. I breathed again, slowing down the moment to absorb every radiant molecule of heat

Summers visiting relatives in Israel, summers spent on warm Mediterranean sands. Summers of heat and humidity punctuated by apricot-flavored ices. Old men lugging ancient iceboxes along the beach. "*Meesh-meesh*," they'd call out for apricot, and I would bound over clutching a silver lira in my fist. Summer evenings spent catching the breeze on the roof of my father's childhood home in the Yemenite quarter of Tel Aviv, squeezed in between the solar heating panels and the creaky water tanks. The *shouk*, the outdoor market, was just at the end of the block. Overripe tomatoes, briny olives, coriander leaves, and frying falafel—their smells would waft over on torpid billows of heat. Fragrant vapors of heat that made me languid with fatigue. Humid exhalations of heat that made the pavement shimmer. Dizzy, drowsy, delicious heat ...

Oh, to be hot. I tore open the prepackaged iodine scrub brush. The brownish-yellow liquid spilled over my hands. I started scrubbing with the stiff plastic brush the way the head nurse had admonished us—fifteen times on the side of my index finger, fifteen times over the fingernail, fifteen times on the other side of the finger. On to the next one. All ten fingers, all the way to the elbows.

Through the glass I could see the patient being prepped. She was a black woman who looked to be in her sixties. I had no idea why she was having a hysterectomy or why her hysterectomy was being done in the middle of the night, but I'd long since given up asking questions on the OB-GYN rotation.

My arms were dripping wet as I backed into the operating room, thumping the door open with my hip as I had been instructed to do. I dripped patiently at the back of the crowd until a nurse was finally free to hand me a sterile towel. She then opened a sterile gown, identical to the one I had been using as a blanket fifteen minutes ago. I slid in and then did the customary whirl so she could tie the strings around my waist. Lastly, I slipped into a pair of sterile gloves—size 6½.

By this point in the month I'd learned to stay out of the way when in the operating room. Everyone was doing important stuff and if I accidentally bumped into a tray, as I had already done twice, I would "unsterilize" all the tools laying on it. The nurse would glare at me and curse under her breath while she unwrapped an entirely new set of sterile equipment. I never did figure out how touching one edge of a three-foot table would instantly unsterilize everything that was on it. It reminded me of "cooties," which spread in a similar manner on my elementary school playground.

I stayed at the edge of the crowd, keeping my hands at shoulder level. I clasped them together in prayer-formation as I had been taught to do to keep from inadvertently unsterilizing them or the surgical tools or the surgical nurse or the surgeon. From the back, I watched the anesthesiologist sedate the woman. He eased an oxygen mask over her face with one hand. The other hand pressed a syringe, discharging medicine into her IV. The patient had finely carved wrinkles that undulated through her dark skin. I saw her lids drift closed over brown eyes.

The operating room was large and stark. Stainless steel shelves and tables shimmered icily, dissipating any possible warmth. Sheets of blue cloth secreted away bundles of sterile instruments, themselves hewn from cold stainless steel. Piercingly bright circles from the lights above the surgical table made the rest of the room appear shaded. In the vast penumbra of the sterile room we were like flitting insects huddling toward the heat and the light.

The patient was now intubated with a breathing tube and lay sound asleep. A blue curtain was raised, sequestering her head from the rest of her body. Only her lower abdomen was exposed. Her belly was a lighter color than her face and it offered the soft buoyancy of many pregnancies. The intern, or maybe it was the second-year resident, dipped gauze in iodine. Beginning in the center, he stroked it in small circles, gradually enlarging them until nearly the whole of the belly was covered in oily brown.

Unusual for a late night operation at Bellevue, there was an attending present. I didn't recognize the attending—I'd never seen him before and his ID card wasn't visible under his gown. By now I was used to being in close quarters with people whose names I didn't know for purposes I didn't understand. And I knew that it wasn't my place to ask. The only thing I could ascertain was that this attending was bearded because he was wearing one of those special surgical hoods that cloaked the hairy jowls that were missed by the standard facemasks. Only his eyes were exposed and they were blurred by large, thick-rimmed glasses.

"You the medical student?" he said to me. I nodded. "Keep your hands where I can see them. I don't want anything contaminated."

I edged in closer so that my hands would be in viewing range for him. The nurse leaned over and murmured to me to place them on the sterile field next to the patient's belly. The blue cloth field contained a scalpel and three metal clamps laid out in parallel next to a neat stack of gauze. I looked at her with a puzzled expression. Why should I put my hands right in the middle of the action? I'd be sure to mess something up that way.

"Do what she says," said the attending. "That's the safest place. Just lay them on the sterile field where I can seem them and they won't get contaminated." I lowered my eyes and did what I was told.

The attending grasped the scalpel and drew a smooth line across the patient's browned lower abdomen. Two edges softly revealed themselves and separated with barely a whisper. Fine rivulets of blood seeped into the chasm. The attending reached in with a pen-sized yellow plastic Bowlby tool. It was the only object in the room that wasn't stainless steel. When he pressed a lever, there was a low buzzing and a trail of smoke wormed its way up out of her belly. The acrid smell of singed flesh seeped into the air and the bleeding ceased.

No matter how many times I've been in an operating room, that pungent cloying smell has never failed to paralyze my senses. Burning skin. Crisping meat. Human sacrifice. Is that how Dachau smelled?

The edges divided, unearthing more flesh—the pink richness of muscle and the oily gold of fat. The attending made his way through the depths, buzzing and separating, cutting and burning. The patient was heavy-set and there were many layers to unveil.

The patient's head was blocked off from my vision with a blue cloth. Every other part of her body was covered. Only the well that was deepening into her belly was exposed.

When I had attended cesarean sections, the dry, boring surgery was at least rewarded by the appearance of a baby. The serious air of the operating room was so easily melted by the wailing bit of infant; everybody had to smile.

But here we were just in a dull operation, chasing down a uterus for reasons that no one had bothered to tell me. In the haze of my mind there was a vague reminder to my body that, according to its biorhythms, it should be asleep. If this were a regular delivery I could convince my body that it was worth it. Babies were always worth it. My first delivery was at the beginning of the month, ages ago when I was still well rested and warm. Joemi was already in labor when I'd shown up at 7:30 that morning. Sanjay, the resident, kept reassuring her, and me, that it would be any minute now. Any minute.

I'd paced the floor, afraid to leave even for the bathroom in case I missed it. Every so often Sanjay would come by and stick a gloved finger into her birth canal. "Almost there," he'd say, with infinite optimism. "Just hang in there."

I attempted to distract Joemi by chatting about medical school and the mayor's plan for a new park on Second Avenue. She tried to be friendly, but labor pains bulldozed over her every few minutes. "Anytime soon," Sanjay sang out at his next brief stopover. "It's coming."

By 4:00 in the afternoon, I could stand my hunger no longer and dashed down to the cafeteria to buy a tuna sandwich. I'd forgotten that 4:00 was "change of shift." The elevator was crammed with day-shift nurses and their bags and their umbrellas, hustling to get out as quickly as possible. And it was packed with evening-shift nurses and their bags and their umbrellas, rushing to get to their posts on time. I tried to protect my lunch from the jostling of the crowd but somebody's backpack swung in my direction and spilled the mound of coleslaw out of its paper saucer. The liquid quickly ran through the paper plate and the pickle slipped precipitously close to the edge. I bent the paper plate in half, trying to create a crevice in the center for everything to slide into, but the coleslaw juice kept dribbling out.

Trying to catch escaping mercury.

"Hey," said the clerk as I walked back into the labor suite with the pickle swimming in the palm of my hand and a small glob of tuna on my white coat, "you the one waiting for that lady to pop? They just took her in a few minutes ago." I threw my soggy plate of tuna on the counter and dashed down the hall to the delivery room. How could this have happened? I'd been waiting all day.

I poked my head in and saw Joemi being prepped. She was semi-reclined on the table and Sanjay was easing her knees apart. "Where've you been?" he called. "I was looking for you everywhere." I started to explain about the coleslaw and the elevator but he cut me off. "You wanna deliver a baby or not? Scrub and get in here, *stat.*"

I kicked on the faucet and realized that the pickle was still in my hand. I slammed it into the garbage pail, leaning over to bury it under some used surgical masks. The scrub brush package fumbled in my hands as I struggled to tear the plastic seal under the pulsing water. How many brush strokes per fingernail? Was I supposed to go thumb to pinky, or was it pinky to thumb? Iodine cascaded over my arms and shirt.

"Step on it," Sanjay yelled. "This babe ain't waiting."

I hurled the scrub brush into the sink and bounded into the room, hoping I didn't smell too much like pickle. A nurse torpedoed me into a gown and gloves while Joemi screamed and clenched at the hand-rails.

"You almost missed it," Sanjay said. "Get in here." Between Joemi's legs a big ball was bulging. "It's crowning, here's your chance." I stepped closer. "Kneel down," he said. Kneel down? "Yeah, yeah, just get on your knees." The two of us knelt on the tile floor and our shoulders were level with Joemi's waist. The ball was getting larger. I could hear Joemi gasping and sputtering as she pushed. "Put out your hands," he ordered. I put out my hands. The ball turned into a little head. A face. Eyes. Nose. A mouth.

"Catch," he said. "Just catch it as it comes out." I held out my hands and a tiny body slithered forth. Sanjay suctioned out the nose and mouth. A chest and arms and legs poured into my hands. He clipped the cord and a high-pitched wail erupted from the liquidy thing in my hands. A baby! A real baby.

"Now get up and carry it over to the nurses," Sanjay said. I wobbled slowly to my feet. "Just don't drop it." I took tiny steps across the gray tile floor—this pink, wet, screaming thing cupped in my hands. Don't drop it, I prayed. There was a clump of blue-gowned nurses in the corner of the delivery room with a warming lamp set up over a small table. So far away, they seemed, stretched way away over the horizon.

I slid my blue booty-clad feet across the floor, afraid that lifting them would unsettle my balance. The baby wriggled in my fingers. I readjusted my palms to catch the round head and rear, but it slithered precariously. Like trying to hold mercury. Please God, don't let me drop it. The piercing shrieks threatened my tenuous balance. I looked back—Sanjay and Joemi were miles behind me, the nurses miles ahead. I stared down at the thing in my hands—it was breathing, coughing, crying. Tiny fingers sporting weensy fingernails flapped about. How could each finger possibly possess a nail that small?

Don't drop it, I prayed. Finally the corner drew near. The baby was whisked from me and plunged into a sea of blue. I stared down at my wet, gloved hands. They had just held a living, breathing infant. They had shepherded it from Joemi's body to the waiting nurses. These hands had actually done something!

Now my hands sat mute. Laid out among the icy silver tools in the sterile field, they were just another part of the dull landscape. A heavy oppressive silence hung over the room, punctuated only by the attending's one-word instrument requests, and the nurse's identical echo.

"Hemostat."

"Hemostat."

Some operating rooms had music. One surgeon was a famous Neil Diamond fan. He would play the same tape over and over during his six-hour heart operations and no one was allowed to change it.

"Ring-tip."

"Ring-tip."

Another attending was a baseball maven. He could recite batting averages and pitching stats for the Yankees but would wax poetic when it came to the Brooklyn Dodgers. "You kids never saw Ebbets Field, didya? We used to climb the trees to watch the games. And '55—oh, '55—that was the last season they grabbed the Series. You kids shoulda been there."

"Metzenbaum."

"Metzenbaum."

Some surgeons loved to "pimp" the students and interns over minute points of anatomy. "What's the origin of the right gastro-epiploic artery?" "What muscle does the ileo-inguinal nerve innervate?" "Describe the peritoneal ligaments that suspend the liver." Those on-the-spot questions tended to unnerve me because I could never come up with the exact distribution of the splenic artery at just that moment, but at least I was learning something.

"Babcock."

"Babcock."

My knees wobbled from fatigue. My whole body cried out to be lying horizontal, under a pile of warm blankets.

"Retractor."

"Retractor."

The attending eased a large red mass out from the well. As the uterus was passed across my line of vision I could see knobby fibroids poking out of the walls.

"5-0 nylon."

"5-0 nylon." Now it was time to sew.

The attending used a tiny curved suture needle secured in the jaws of a bulky metal clamp. He held the clamp in his hand like a pair of pliers. In and out of the well the clamp sailed, a thin black strand of silk trailing behind. After the thread ran out, the attending plunked the heavy clamp down and demanded another. The nurse scurried to set a fresh needle and thread in a new clamp, but she couldn't seem to keep up with his rapid suturing.

Plunk. "Another 5-0. Can I get another 5-0?" I saw the nurse's eyes flash back and forth.

"5-0," she said, passing him another clamp.

My feet were growing numb from standing in one position. My eyelids were drooping.

Plunk. "5-0."

"5-0."

What gain could there possibly be from my presence in this operating room? I wasn't helping anyone and I wasn't learning anything. I could feel my body wavering, crying out its desire to be horizontal.

Plunk. Sting

My fingers jolted awake. Something bit me. Something stung me. I looked down to my hands sitting in their place on the sterile field. A clamp with its needle lay askew next to my index finger. A tiny black speck marked its breech of my glove.

I'd been stuck. My breath caught in my throat. I'd been stuck with a needle.

"Suction."

"Suction."

I looked toward the nurse. She caught my eyes briefly then glanced away. I looked toward the attending. I saw the tail end of his gaze returning to his suturing. He must have seen it. He must have. How could he not? I scanned the faces around me. Mouths and noses were covered up. Hair and foreheads were veiled. Expressions were buried in layers of sterile cotton. Just eyes poking through. Only eyes. But I couldn't decipher what any of the eyes were saying.

But a needle! I'd just been stuck by a needle.

My hands lay frozen on the sterile field next to the clamp. My breath remained frozen in my throat. My eyes roamed blindly through the heavy air, but there was nothing to see.

"Sponge."

"Sponge."

Was I allowed to speak? Did third-year medical students have that right? I'd never been stuck before. If the attending wasn't saying anything then it probably wasn't that important. If the nurse wasn't saying anything then this must be a routine part of surgery. If everyone is silent then this must be the way it goes.

Finally someone announced that the operation was over. I dashed out of the room and tore off my gloves. There was a tiny prick in my right index finger—small as a pencil mark, but it was there. I wrenched on the faucet full force and plunged my hand into the burning water. Who was that patient? What if she had AIDS? I squeezed my finger, trying to force blood out—my blood, her blood, tainted blood. I wanted it out.

The hot water seared my skin and I cursed the burning heat. I squeezed my skin harder, blanching it under the steaming water. I tore open a bottle of iodine and disgorged it over my finger, the inky brown cascading down into the drain. Out, out, I implored. Get out.

The operating room had emptied. The patient had been wheeled to recovery and the nurses and doctors had dispersed to wherever nurses and doctors go in the middle of the night. Where was everybody? Only frigid stainless steel remained in the room.

I walked back to the call room, the lonely room with the rancid mattress on the floor. I crawled onto the mattress, under the coarse paper gown that was my blanket. The dimness was oddly comforting after the bright lights of the operating room. Is that it, I wondered. Years of studying and struggling, and then one little needle stick and it's all over? How could it be that simple? I wanted to think more, to think harder, but my mind couldn't unglue from its frozen muddle. Mercury frozen in mid-spill—chaos preserved in ice. I pulled the paper gown higher over me to keep the shivers and the tears at bay.

∽I woke up later, unclear if it had been hours or days. The room was dim even though the lights were on. It was cold. There were no windows, no clocks, no indications of day or night. Where was I?

I stumbled out the door, rubbing my eyes. Slowly, it came back. Bellevue. Medical student. OB-GYN. Overnight call. Midnight surgery. Needle stick.

I looked down at my hand. The tiny black mark on my right index finger was still there.

A needle stick! My stomach awoke with a start, churning its panicked insistence at me. My cheeks began to quiver. I've got to do something, fast. What?

Stay calm. Act like a real doctor. Just go over and read her chart. You were at the surgery, you're entitled to read the chart. Find out her history before you panic. Maybe she's already been tested and is negative. Maybe there's nothing at all to worry about. If not, just go talk to the patient. Ask her if she would take an HIV test. I supposed that was what a real doctor would do.

I bit my teeth down hard. And pursed my lips for good measure.

I walked over to the desk where the surgery list was posted and scanned for the overnight operations. Angeline Burton was the only hysterectomy listed. Room 9E23.

I gingerly pulled out Angeline Burton's chart. It was pink, like all the other charts in the OB-GYN division. In the rest of the hospital the charts were blue. I ran my hand over the rough plastic covers of the notebook, tracing the letters of her name. What if the chart said she was an IV drug user? What if the chart said she had hepatitis? What if the chart said she lived on the street?

I hesitated with the pink cover in my hand. This chart with Mrs. Burton's history could hold my destiny, my life. I had not taken her history in the traditional sense of a doctor interviewing a patient, but I felt I was about to take her history in a far more profound manner—I was going to absorb her history. Her history could now become my history. Her blood my blood. Her story mine.

I turned to the admitting history. "Chief complaint: Patient is a sixty-seven-year-old female admitted for bleeding fibroids." So far, so good. "Past Medical History: diabetes requiring insulin, hypertension." Good, diabetes and hypertension—nice healthy diseases. "Social History: born in Virginia. No history of tobacco, alcohol, or drugs." Whew, no drugs. Good Southern background. But who ever tells the truth to doctors when asked about drugs. "Widowed, four children. Lives with eldest daughter." Okay, sounds tame enough. "Retired. Worked as nurse at Bronx Lebanon Hospital for thirty-four years."

Nurse? Bronx Lebanon? That's it, I was sunk. A nurse. She'd probably gotten a million needle sticks in her thirty-four years of work. For sure she'd gotten exposed to AIDS. And if not AIDS, then at least hepatitis. Two hundred health care workers died every year from hepatitis B, I'd been told. And now there was hepatitis C. I scanned the chart for any signs of an HIV test, but there were none.

That's how they'd tell my story. Promising medical student, they'd say, till she got that needle stick. A nurse from Bronx Lebanon, they'd cluck, shaking their heads. Hep B, Hep C, AIDS—that lady had everything. And less than a year from graduation, what a shame. They named a bench after her in the Bellevue park.

Stay calm, I told myself as I started down the hall. You can handle this. Just go to her room and ask her for an HIV test. It's very simple. Forget the idiot attending and just go straight to the patient; that's the way a real doctor would handle it. And you're becoming a doctor, right?

Angeline Burton lay in her bed with the headrest raised high up so that she was nearly sitting. She was a portly woman with large breasts that settled over her ample belly. Crinkly gray hair with bits of black poking through was pinned behind her ears. She stared out the window toward the river. A meal tray consisting of only liquids sat next to her bed, untouched. There was a Bible and a small picture of a glowing Jesus perched next to the can of ginger ale. A small bouquet of yellow daisies on the windowsill was on the verge of wilting, but hadn't yet.

I tiptoed into the room and cleared my throat quietly. "Mrs. Burton?" She turned her head quickly at the sound of my voice and soft brown eyes settled on mine. I took a half step back. "I ... I'm sorry to disturb you. I know you are resting...."

"No, honey," she broke into an easy smile. "It's all right. I'm just staring at the water, that's all. It's so pretty when the sun rises, don't you think?"

I followed her gaze out the window to where the industrial plants of Queens hovered across the East River. The early morning sunlight lent a soft glimmer even to the smokestacks. The river itself was almost blinding in its brightness. I nodded.

"I ... I'm one of the medical students who was at your surgery last night."

"You were? How nice of you to visit me. So few of the doctors ever come around to see you in this place. It's so nice to see a pretty young face in the morning."

"Well ... I ..."

"These hospitals can be lonely places for patients. Emily—that's my daughter—she came visited me yesterday, but she couldn't get off work for today. The phone company where she works at is real strict about days off. And she's used so many up with Denise's asthma attacks. Every day, it seems, there's another attack. She's always hauling that girl to the doctor. I used to take care of Denise whenever she got them attacks, but my diabetes has gotten bad and my feet just ain't the way they used to be."

She stopped suddenly and put a hand to her mouth. "Dear me, I'm sorry honey, blabbering off like that. I bet you come on medical business and here's me going on about Denise's asthma attacks. I know you ain't interested in Denise and her asthma."

"I came to, uh, talk to you about your surgery." I swallowed hard to keep my voice even. The swallow started my cheeks quivering.

"I am sure glad to get that over and done with. I been dreading that operation for weeks. Every time my doctor said I should get it done I wouldn't listen to her. Too much to think about. But the bleeding and the aches—they really came on something fierce lately. So I came round and finally did it." She adjusted the tape on the IV fixed into her arm. "And you know what? It wasn't so bad after all. I mean, once I was asleep it was like magic. I seen people go into surgery lots of times, but it ain't the same when you're the one on the stretcher."

AIDS. Hepatitis B. Hepatitis C.

"Mrs. Burton?" I started again.

"Yes, honey. What can I do for you?"

"Mrs. Burton? I ... I wanted to ask ..."

"If it's about the insurance, don't worry, 'cause Emily did of all the Medicare papers and I do have retirement coverage from my job."

"No, no. It's not that." The trembling started to spread over my entire face. "I wanted to ask you ..."

"Something the matter?" She looked at me, her eyes crinkling with concern. "Did they find something bad at the operation? Is that it?"

I shook my head, pressing my teeth against my lips.

"'Cause if it is, you can tell me. I may look like an old lady, but I'm pretty strong."

I shook my head again, but this time my lips began to quiver.

"You okay, honey? You look a little peaked." She patted the edge of the bed. "Sit. Come sit down."

I took the seat hesitantly, remembering an attending who had admonished us never to sit on a patient's bed. It's condescending and an invasion of privacy, he'd told us. I wanted to act professional. I wanted to handle this like a real doctor, not a measly medical student, but the spot on the bed looked so inviting. The sheets were comfortably mussed from sleep. When I sat down, the trembling worsened.

"What's up, honey?" Mrs. Burton touched her fingertips to my arm. They were warm. "You look like something's got you."

I nodded and sucked in my breath. "Mrs. Burton, last night ... last night, during the operation, it was late ..." I paused, determined to keep my tears out of this. I was going to do this like a doctor, not like a little kid. "Last night, it was late and one of the needles ... one of the needles stuck my finger. It stuck me." The sobs were pressing forward but I sniffled them back. "I got stuck."

"Oh, honey," Mrs. Burton said, drawing out her words slowly and softly, "that must have really hurt."

I nodded, holding on as best I could. "I wanted to ask you ..."

"What's on your mind, honey?" Her fingers encircled my arm and the warmth spread.

"You know," I sniffled, "all those, you know, diseases...."

"Diseases?"

"Those diseases, like uh," I swallowed dryly, "like AIDS and stuff."

"Oh," she said with a chuckle. "I thought you were talking about my diabetes. You don't need to worry about no diseases with me." Her arms slid easily over mine. The undersides were surprisingly smooth.

"But you were a nurse," I said, the tears trembling at the edges. "A nurse ..."

"It's okay," she whispered. "It's okay." She pulled me forward gently. Before I knew it, I had sunk into her arms crying. The soft heat of her chest brought my sobs on even harder.

"At Bronx Lebanon . . ." I blubbered.

"Shhhh," she said. "It's okay. I know what you're saying." She rubbed her hand in circles along my back, pressing deeper and deeper into the muscles.

"And needle sticks . . . you must have gotten so many needle sticks."

"You don't have nothing to worry about me, honey," she said softly. "I was a nurse's aide. I didn't handle no needles or nothing—that was for the LPNs and the RNs. Besides, they made us do all those tests for our annual employee physicals. I came out fine every year." Her other hand supported the back of my head. I could feel her fingers running through the tangles of my hair. The muscles of my neck unraveled to her touch. "And my Samuel, may God bless his soul, he's been gone nearly fifteen years now. You don't have nothing to worry about."

"I'm sorry, Mrs. Burton. I didn't want to . . ."

"Shhh, it's okay, honey. I know you're scared. Everybody is." Her fingers spread to encompass my entire back. "It's okay."

I sobbed in her arms and she held me tight. I didn't feel anything like what I thought a real doctor should be feeling. A real doctor wouldn't be weeping in her patient's arms.

I cried until I was drained. Maybe I even dozed, I don't know. But when I uncurled myself from Mrs. Burton and stood up, I felt as though I had slept a whole night and was already onto a new day. I blinked my eyes to gather my bearings. Mrs. Burton was smiling at me.

"You go, honey, and be a good doctor." She reached over and squeezed my hand. "God be watching over you and you'll be fine. See, he's making that sun shine right now for you." She nodded toward the East River. "It's a day from heaven just waiting for you to go out and kiss it."

I couldn't get any words out, but the numbness in my legs had finally dissipated. The tightness in my head had at last softened. For the first time in weeks I felt unmuddled. The slithering mercury had been scooped back together, restored to its order and stashed safely away. I squeezed her hand in return and tried to memorize her brown eyes. Then I left her arms. I left the room. I left the hallway. I left the ward. I left Bellevue and went out to kiss the day.

CHAPTER FOUR

Change of Heart

My ideal doctor would be my Virgil, leading me through my purgatory or inferno, pointing out the sights as we go . . . He would see the genius of my illness. He would mingle his daemon with mine; we would wrestle with my fate together. Inside every patient, there's a poet trying to get out. My ideal doctor would "read" my poetry, my literature.

Anatole Broyard, "Doctor, Talk to Me"

SUB-INTERNSHIP is the one chance a medical student gets to really "play doctor." Now that I had completed all the third-year clerkships— medicine, surgery, OB-GYN, pediatrics, psychiatry, and neurology—I was entitled, as a fourth-year medical student, to a year's worth of electives plus six weeks of sub-internship. As a "sub," medical students assumed the full responsibilities of an intern, including all patient care, all scut, all on-call. Technically, two medical students were supposed to fill the role of one intern—the theory being that two sub-interns equal one intern—but in practice, usually only one sub was assigned to each intern position. As such, you were a full-fledged member of the team, admitting the same number of patients as a regular intern. It's the first time you didn't feel absolutely obliged to correct someone when they called you doctor.

The Manhattan VA where I had been assigned was populated mainly by WWII veterans suffering from lung cancer and heart disease, but there were the "youngsters" from Korea and Vietnam who brought in drug abuse and AIDS. The VA still possessed open wards —cavernous rooms lined with metal-framed beds. There were sixteen beds to a room, separated by long pale blue curtains that dangled from the high ceilings. The advantages of the VA over Bellevue—the

"Va-Spa" vs. "the Vue"—could be summed up by two things, according to my more knowledgeable classmates: the patients spoke English and the staircases were unlocked.

I had finished my third-year rotations and now I was officially a fourth-year student. But my fourth year of medical school was only to last these six weeks of sub-internship. My research and doctoral dissertation didn't conform to the neatly organized medical school calendar and therefore had started me in the wrong place as a third-year. The only way to graduate within the expected seven years of the MD-PhD program was to forgo all the cushy fourth-year electives (dermatology in San Francisco, endocrine in Puerto Rico) and just do the required sub. Six weeks as a sub-intern and then I would graduate medical school.

I hoped I would instantly acquire a swagger in my walk once I became a fourth-year medical student. My new long white coat looked just like the ones the interns wore, distinct from the short, boxy coat I'd been wearing all year as a third-year. I'd grown to hate that short coat, which screamed to the world just how inexperienced I was. Now I was wearing the coat that was the length of a real doctor. (Of course the "School of Medicine" insignia was a dead giveaway to anyone who came close, as was my ID card). From a distance, however, I could potentially be mistaken for an intern or resident . . . even, perhaps, an attending.

On my first day as a sub one of the interns took me to the supply room and helped stuff my pockets with intern paraphernalia: 16, 18, and 20 gauge IVs ("20s for meds and fluids, 18s for blood, 16s if they're really crashing"—I had already figured out that smaller numbers meant larger sizes, but I never understood why), a roll of surgical tape, 4x4 sterile gauze pads, assorted syringes, alcohol swabs, speckle-top blood tubes, and butterfly needles. He even gave me a drug-company pen. I tried to arrange my equipment as Li-Chan had, tucking my supplies into various pockets, clipping the roll of tape onto the side slit. All I needed was a gleaming silver barrette to hook into my buttonhole. Suddenly a mysterious sound arose from my waistline, a crackly voice mumbling something unintelligible. My beeper! My beeper was going off. I was being paged!

I stared at the metal box affixed to my belt. A real beeper! Somebody was actually paging me. A flower of emotion unfurled inside of me and crept through my body, but I couldn't quite identify it. Awe? Pride? Simple glee? It was as though I had been pushed up over the next precipice and was now on higher ground with sweeter crisper mountain air to breathe. Somebody was paging me. Somebody needed me. I had a purpose.

After a few minutes the other intern nudged me. "You have to answer the page," he said gently. "You probably have an admission."

Herbert Ziff's chart arrived on 12-South before he did. He was a "frequent flier" at the VA owing to his continued IV drug use, and the heft of his medical record accurately reflected that. His heart valves repeatedly became infected with endocarditis, each time necessitating up to six weeks in the hospital for antibiotics. On several occasions, fragments of bacteria-infested tissue escaped from his heart and sailed along to other body parts, lodging in his kidney, brain, and legs. The CT scan of his head showed two golf-ball size scars where the infection had eaten away portions of the frontal lobe of his brain. "Frontal lobe syndrome," my resident Miguel commented. "Disinhibited."

Mr. Ziff also had HIV. His T-cells, however, were only a bit below normal. So far he had not experienced any HIV-related infections. He wasn't even on any HIV medications.

"This gentleman is quite lucky in the T-cell department," Miguel said. "His immune system is nearly normal." Miguel, like so many of the VA housestaff, was an "FMG"—a foreign medical graduate. The term FMG was tossed around a lot in the medical community, often in a derogatory manner. Community hospitals in rural areas tended to be staffed by FMGs, with the unspoken undertone that no graduate of a red-blooded American medical school would ever want to work in places of such low prestige. It was apparently difficult for FMGs to gain positions at larger medical centers. Later on I learned that if it weren't for the FMGs, there would be almost no medical care in small community hospitals in most of America, but no one ever mentioned that.

Miguel had been raised in upper-middle class Venezuela. He'd attended private Catholic schools and the most prestigious college and medical school. He'd completed an entire medical residency in South America but was now repeating it in New York in order to apply to competitive American cardiology fellowships. For him, life in the hospital was old-hat. Nothing fazed or unnerved him, which was a relief to me, for whom everything was a potential land mine. He enjoyed sharing his knowledge and never minded when the other members of the team made fun of his throaty accent. He was more well-read in European and American literature than I was, and he was as likely to expound upon Flaubert as he was upon hypokalemia.

Mr. Ziff lay asleep on his bed with his left hand in his underwear when Miguel and I approached him. He was a skinny black fellow who appeared much younger than his forty-three years. He awoke with a smile when I shook his shoulder.

"Mornin' to you, Doc, Doc" he said, acknowledging each of us individually. "Pleasure to be here." There was a childlike sweetness to his smile.

I waited for Miguel to begin taking the history as all my other residents had, but he nudged me and nodded. I was a sub now—I had to do it on my own.

"Nice to meet you, Mr. Ziff," I said, and then my mind went entirely blank. I stared down at my clipboard, hoping to remember something, anything, that I was supposed to ask when taking a medical history. I could so clearly visualize the silvery-gray cover of my *History and Physical* textbook, but I couldn't think of one single word from the inside. All I could remember was the logo on the front cover. Miguel leaned over and whispered, "Chief complaint."

Chief complaint, of course. "So Mr. Ziff," I said, swallowing and adjusting my voice to its most doctorly tone, "what brings you to the hospital today?" That was how I'd recalled my residents fishing out the chief complaint.

"This time I come by ambulance. Last time my wife brought me."

Miguel chuckled quietly. I pressed on. "I mean, why did you decide to come to the hospital? What symptoms did you have?" I noticed that the hand that was tucked in his shorts had started to move about.

"Doc, I just wasn't feeling too good. You know, fevers and all. Breathing's been a little heavy these days. My wife took me to Cornell, but after they see I was a veteran, they send me by ambulance over here. But that's okay, I been here before and I like the food." He paused and looked at me with wide eyes. "You ever been to the Brooklyn VA? Don't ever! The food ain't good enough for pigs." Then he smiled impishly. "But here they know how to do it right."

Past medical history. "Have you ever been sick before, Mr. Ziff?"

"Shoot, yeah, I been sick before. I been in the Albany VA, the Philadelphia VA, and in one of them VAs over in Jersey. Can't remember the name, but they sure had nice lookin' social workers."

Mr. Ziff's answers to my questions were a bit spotty, but he gamely offered a convoluted journey through family history, social history, and review of systems. Miguel and I then set him up for an EKG. When we ran the machine there was too much background muscle activity from his left arm. I asked him to hold still for one minute so we could get a clean EKG tracing. "Sure, Doc," Mr. Ziff said, like a child trying his best to obey the teacher. But his hand kept going and the EKG was illegible.

I asked him again to hold still. "It's okay, Doc, I'm not moving a muscle!" Mr. Ziff said brightly. His arm kept churning and the EKG slid all over the page. "Do you know what time they bring the lunch trays around here?"

"Frontal lobe syndrome," Miguel muttered, reddening a bit near his ears.

A nurse came in to provide assistance. She put her hands on her hips and looked sternly at Mr. Ziff. "Now Herbert, don't you do that in front of the nice lady doctor."

Mr. Ziff grinned at her. "Sure thing, honey, I promise." I couldn't help but smile at his earnestness. The nurse finally pinned his left arm

down to minimize the gyrations while I obtained a close approxima-
tion of an EKG.

When I finished, there was a long strip of wobbly tracings in my
hand. I began to wind the EKG leads around the machine. "Hey Doc,"
Mr. Ziff said, his gaze gentle and trusting. "I really 'preciate all you're
doing for me. They got good doctors here at the VA, I know that. I
would never take my body anyplace else." He nodded, his voice tinged
with an innocence. "You're going to be my doc, right?"

I took a small step backward involuntarily. It was the first time anyone had ever referred to me as a doctor, as *their* doctor. "I ... I guess so.
I'm going to be your doctor," I said. I tucked the EKG bulbs under the
handle of the cart and felt a soft flush warming inside my chest. Somebody actually considered me their doctor.

As I wheeled the EKG cart out of the room he called out, "Say, Doc,
do you think when you're writing them orders you could be so kind as
to order me double portions on the meals?"

"Don't worry, Mr. Ziff," I said, a bit more confidently now. "I'll take
care of you."

✐The next day we gathered for morning report, the daily case conference in the Department of Medicine. Dr. Weber, the chief of medicine, sat in the middle of the front row, flanked by several other senior
attendings. The chief residents sat in the second row. Behind them
were all the other residents, interns, sub-interns, and medical students.
The interns who had worked overnight were slumped in the back, already asleep.

"This morning we'll be discussing the case of Mr. Herbert Ziff," the
chief resident announced, reading from a green ledger. "Will the doctor who admitted Mr. Ziff please give the presentation."

Hmmm, I thought. Mr. Ziff's case must really be important. I leaned
back in my chair with my cup of coffee, proud that my patient's case
was going to be discussed, and proud that my resident was going to
speak in front of the whole department.

"Herbert Ziff?" the chief resident called out again. "The doctor taking care of Mr. Ziff?"

Miguel elbowed me in the ribs. "That's you."

"Me?" I nearly spit out my coffee onto his white coat. "I don't have any of my notes with me."

I hedged my way forward to the lectern and grabbed onto the edges to steady myself. There was a sea of white coats and white Styrofoam coffee cups in front of me. Dr. Weber was front and center. He was a portly man with a ruddy, fleshy face topped with a few stray tufts of white hair. In another setting he might have been described as jolly, but here he was buttoned up in a stiff white coat with a severe expression on his face. His stocky arms were crossed tightly in front of him.

I took a deep breath and leaned hard on the lectern. Chief complaint. "Mr. Ziff is a forty-three-year-old male." Was his chief complaint shortness of breath, or swelling of his legs?

Past medical history. "The patient has a long history of IV drug use and multiple episodes of endocarditis." Did the brain abscess come before the kidney infection, or did the kidney infection occur with his first bout of endocarditis? Dr. Weber sat expressionless, staring straight at me.

Miguel motioned slightly with his hand. His lips were moving in pantomime. I strained forward to make out what he was saying. "Physical exam," he mouthed silently.

I cleared my throat. "Physical exam. On physical exam the patient was a thin black male. He was short of breath and he had a loud heart murmur." Was it a systolic murmur or a diastolic murmur? Crescendo or decrescendo?

Miguel crooked his finger and pointed quietly to his stomach.

"Abdomen. His abdomen was soft, non-tender, non-distended."

I struggled through the physical exam and then I paused, not sure what came next. Dr. Weber held out a thick-fingered hand. "EKG, please."

I fished around in my pocket, sifting through the IVs, alcohol pads, and assorted blood tubes, until I extracted the crumpled roll of EKG paper. I smoothed it out and deposited it into the waiting hand. The room was silent as Dr. Weber examined the EKG. I shuffled my position at the lectern.

Dr. Weber frowned, stringing the three-foot strip through his hands. His eyes zigzagged back and forth over the pink graph paper and his forehead contracted into ever-deeper furrows. Finally he held it up. "This EKG is uninterpretable," he pronounced to the audience. "I expect the housestaff to make better efforts to produce valid data."

"Well," I stammered, "I did try a few times, but this was the best I could get."

"This," he raised his hand up, the strip of wobbling lines dangling from his palm,"was the best you could do?"

"The patient was." I paused, thinking of Mr. Ziff's innocent smile. "... moving. He was moving a lot."

"Even the most restless patient can hold still for the one minute it takes to do an EKG," Dr. Weber said, shaking his head with a sputter.

"The patient was ... occupied." I could see Miguel begin to blush.

"Occupied?"

"Yes sir. Mr. Ziff, was, uh, self-occupied." A few snickers arose from the audience.

"Self-occupied?"

I bit my lip, focusing on the fake wood grain of the lectern. "With his privates, sir," I whispered.

℘Mr. Ziff settled into the VA routine. He smoked regularly in the lounge with all the other veterans. He had somehow obtained a wheelchair and was forever zooming about the halls in his "Z-mobile," comfortably attired in his maroon and green VA-issued pajamas.

"Hey Doc," he would say with his goofy grin, slamming to a halt in front of me. "I need that morphine. This ol' body of mine aches all over." I was never sure if he really had pain or was just seeking drugs. But he was always pleasant and sweet-tempered. And every morning on rounds we would come upon him, sound asleep with a gentle smile on his face, his hand planted firmly in his underwear.

Mr. Ziff's biggest problem was his heart valve. It had been ravaged by so many infections that it now just billowed helplessly as his blood surged by. The resulting heart murmur was so loud that one almost did not need a stethoscope to hear it. His blood sloshed recklessly through his arteries and it was possible to run a hand down his calf and trace the pulse of blood as it moved. Mr. Ziff was so skinny, and his aortic valve so helpless, that one could actually see the ripples of blood coursing through his body, all the way down to his toes. Troops of medical students came by to observe the classic signs of aortic insufficiency.

Mr. Ziff needed a new valve. Indeed, he had been scheduled for an aortic valve replacement twice in the past, but each time he returned to using IV drugs and the surgery was canceled. When I asked him about it, he would shrug with a resigned smile. "You know how it happens, Doc. I get clean for a bit, but then there's such good shit on the street. It just happens."

At some point, Herbert Ziff's valve would fail completely. Blood would flood his lungs and he would die instantly if he weren't fortunate enough to be in a hospital at that exact moment for emergency surgery. "But this time, Doc," he said, "I'm staying clean. No more shit for me. My wife and my daughter need me around." He clapped his hand over his chest. "I gotta get this heart back on track."

"It's really important, Mr. Ziff," I said. "Your life is at stake."

"You got it right, Doc. I be telling the boys in the street, 'Ol' Z-man is clean now.'" He gave me a grin and I could see the gaps where his teeth used to be. "You know Doc, you sound like what my wife used to say. She used to tell me all the time, 'Herbert, this stuff's no good for you.' But I ain't always listen. But today's a new day. Yessir, ol' Z-man is clean."

I smiled back. "It sounds like you're ready to get things together. I'm really impressed."

"Yeah, I can do it. It's no problem. Say listen, my bones be aching real bad. That Tylenol with codeine don't do nothing for these old bones." Mr. Ziff pointed out the craggy ulcers that had formed near the tattoos on his legs. "Doc, you think you can give something with a little more umph to it? There ain't no way I can do no drug rehab with my bones aching the way they are." He cocked his head and let loose that grin again. "You know how it is, Doc."

. . .

✑Miguel instructed me to discuss Mr. Ziff's case with the cardiac surgeons so we could start the preparation for a new valve. It took me nearly a week to track them down. I finally caught up with the team striding from the operating room toward the surgical ward. They were dressed in blue scrubs with matching blue shower-cap hats. Blue booties covered their clogs, which clomped loudly as they pressed down the hall. I read to them from my notes, shuffling the pages in order to get the pertinent facts out quickly as I galloped to keep up with them. They looked at each other and nearly burst out laughing. "You want us to operate on him? He'll just shoot up again and destroy the new valve. Besides, he has HIV. That'll kill him anyway. It's not worth it."

"But he has a very high T-cell count and isn't likely to die from AIDS just yet." I was getting winded trying to walk and talk and think at the same time. "And he's promised to give up drugs completely this time."

"And you believe him?" they said with a snort. They clomped off to the surgical ward, leaving me standing with my fistful of notes.

✑Mr. Ziff kept mentioning a wife and a daughter, but I'd never seen them. Most patients at the VA had few, if any, visitors. I simply assumed that he was making it up, or telling me about a past family that had long since abandoned him. He looked and spoke like someone who'd been living on the streets for years, shooting up and sleeping in abandoned buildings. One day, however, I walked into his room and there were two women sitting by his bed as he slept. The older one wore a teal green suit with a floral scarf. Her matching hat was wide brimmed and sported cloth flowers. The younger one was a teenager. She wore jeans and a sweater, and a backpack was slung over her shoulder. The older woman stood up when I entered. Her voice was rich and velvety. "Hello Dr. Ofri. I'm Mrs. Ziff and this is Desiree."

"I'm not his actual doct..." I started, and then stopped. For Mr. Ziff and his family, I was his doctor. I straightened up and held out my hand. "Nice to meet you." The soft flush returned inside my chest.

"Herbert has told us all about you," Mrs. Ziff continued. "We're so glad to finally meet you." She put her hand on her husband's shoulder and rubbed gentle circles. Mr. Ziff stirred and started to awaken. "I know we don't get to visit too often—it's a bus then two subways from Queens—but I'm glad we got to meet you this time."

Desiree walked to the other side of the bed. She took his hand. "Hi Daddy. It's me."

"How's my baby? How's my Desiree?" Mr. Ziff said, his sleep fading and a gap-toothed smile growing.

"I'm good, Daddy. I'm good."

"How you doing in school? You passing all your classes?"

"I'm doing okay."

Mrs. Ziff straightened her hat and announced, "Desiree just won a runner-up award at the science fair."

Mr. Ziff pulled his other arm over and clasped Desiree's hand between his two palms. "You did that, baby? You won an award at the science fair?"

Desiree smiled, her cheeks glowing amber. "Yes, Daddy. I did."

Mr. Ziff looked at me, beaming. "You hear that, Doc? My baby won a science award. My baby won an award."

The days and weeks went by. Mr. Ziff's infection stabilized but his leaky heart valve was a time bomb. On his bad days he would be too short of breath to walk more than a few steps. I kept pestering the cardiac surgeons about a valve replacement. They were adamant in their refusal to operate. Mr. Ziff's story filtered its way through the hospital hierarchy. One day I was informed that an ethics committee was being convened to discuss the case of Herbert Ziff.

"An ethics committee?" Miguel said. "I've been at this VA for three years and I've never seen or heard of any ethics committee."

On Monday morning I arrived in the conference room on the twelfth floor carrying stacks of notes. It was the same room in which I'd presented Mr. Ziff's case to Dr. Weber. The chairs had now been arranged in a circle. A psychiatrist with a specialty in medical ethics was chairing the meeting. He was flanked on either side by two other members of the ethics committee. The head nurse from 12-South was there, as was Mr. Ziff's social worker. A counselor from the drug rehab program had been invited in addition to the chaplain. I recognized one of the surgical residents slurping from a cup of coffee, the strings of his surgical mask dangling dangerously close to the opening on the lid. Next to him was a surgical attending, Dr. Reskin. Both surgeons were wearing regulation blue scrubs.

Dr. Reskin carried with him a battered leather briefcase that was legendary in the medical center. That briefcase must have been more than twenty years old. The original brown or burgundy or black leather had long since faded away to a generic grayish hue. The handles had frayed, the zipper was broken, papers were always falling out of the cracks, but Dr. Reskin would never be parted from that briefcase. It was rumored that he never trifled with, or even noticed, the small-fry of the hospital hierarchy, which probably included everyone from medical students to chief residents, even junior attendings. It was amazing that he'd even condescended to show up at our little meeting.

I slid into a free seat next to the social worker, trying to keep my notes from sliding out of Mr. Ziff's chart. She winked at me, and I tried to smile back but the muscles around my mouth were too tight with nervousness.

The psychiatrist was a gentleman in his seventies, tall and thin with heavily chiseled features. He wore a tweed jacket with leather patches at the elbows and one slender gold pen peeking out from the breast pocket. Bushy eyebrows tufted over his eyes, casting scholarly shadows across his face. He stroked his nonexistent beard a few times, then cleared his throat. "Thank you all for taking the time out of your busy schedules for this meeting. The ethics committee doesn't visit the VA too frequently, but it is an honor to be here." He pulled a scrap of paper out from his jacket pocket. "Today we are here to discuss the case of Herbert Ziff. We encourage everyone to voice their opinions. The committee will then meet over the course of the next two weeks and render a decision. Let me remind you that we are here in the best interest of the patient. That should be in the forefront of our minds." He stuffed the paper back into his pocket. "We'll begin with a brief review of the case by the medical doctor."

There was a long pause and nobody spoke. Then I realized that there was no one else from the Department of Medicine in the room. The surgeons certainly weren't going to present the case. I was Mr. Ziff's doctor. I quickly flipped the chart open and pulled out my notes.

"Mr. Herbert Ziff is a forty-three-year-old gentleman who has had many heart valve infections," I said. "His aortic valve is very weak and needs to be replaced, otherwise he is at risk for sudden death."

The surgical resident interrupted before I could get any further in the medical history. "Listen, I don't want to sound like the bad guy, but let's be realistic. Mr. Ziff has never spent any significant time in his life off drugs. This is a long and complicated operation. It will probably cost ten thousand dollars, which he can never pay. And then he'll just shoot up again and ruin the valve. He'll be back here for a new valve in no time at all. What is the point of putting in all of our time and energy?"

"I know he's used drugs a lot in the past, but this time is different," I insisted. "He truly feels the symptoms of his valve problem—he is short of breath, he can barely walk. I think he realizes now that his life is at stake."

"Come on, how can you believe him?" The resident clamped the cover back on to his coffee. "You know these drug users, they'll say anything you want to hear. That's how they survive on the street."

"Mr. Ziff is different than other drug users, though. He has a wife and a daughter. They can help him stay off drugs."

The members of the ethics committee jumped into the discussion with gusto. Issues flew back and forth across the room as they argued whether a utilitarian model versus a beneficence model would be the better paradigm for this ethical dilemma. Fiduciary relations competed with nonmaleficence, third-party interests battled with patient autonomy. Some quoted Kant, others Locke.

The surgical resident had slipped a scut sheet out from his pocket and was surreptitiously reviewing his upcoming day's work. He slumped further in his seat and I could see that he was growing impatient with all of this academic palaver. He leaned slightly toward Dr.

Reskin. "Not to mention his HIV…" he said out of the side of his mouth.

I was prepared for this and broke back into the discussion. "HIV presents a challenge to all of us in the medical profession," I said, trying to choose words that sounded professional and learned. "Even though these patients have an ultimately fatal disease, they still deserve the highest standard of care. We, as physicians, cannot abandon our patients with HIV. Besides, Mr. Ziff's HIV is not very advanced and I personally do not think it is clinically relevant to his current need for a valve." I nodded my head curtly and closed the chart on my lap. It was true, Mr. Ziff's HIV was not very advanced right now, but I knew, as probably did everyone else in the room, that HIV meant certain death. In the days before protease inhibitors and multidrug therapy, HIV could run a rapid course.

Dr. Reskin spoke now. His voice was gruff and he looked like he hadn't shaved in three days. "It's very easy for you to say that he deserves a valve no matter what his HIV status is, but you're not the one who will be up to your elbows in his HIV-positive blood for five hours." He pushed back some of the unruly hair that had slipped out from under his surgical cap. "I put myself and my entire team at great risk to do this operation. What if somebody gets cut during the procedure? What if some young resident contracts HIV from operating on this guy who doesn't even care about his own life? What am I supposed to tell them when they get AIDS?"

A silence seeped over the group. I looked down at my hands, staring at the finger that had gotten stuck during Angeline Burton's hysterectomy. I shuddered, remembering the terror of thinking that my whole life might have changed from that one event. That tiny moment in time potentially could have multiplied out and dominated the rest of my life.

Nobody spoke. The psychiatrist finally moved to close the meeting. He thanked us for attending and said the committee would meet again to continue the discussion.

. . .

∽A week later I finished my sub-internship, and with that, my seven years of medical school. Graduation was sweet. In the morning was the big NYU commencement in Washington Square Park in Greenwich Village. The entire graduating class of the university crammed into the park. Streets were closed off to accommodate the crowds. The chamber orchestra played from on top of the famous Washington Square Arch at the foot of Fifth Avenue. In the afternoon was the private medical school ceremony in Carnegie Hall with a reception at the Plaza Hotel near the entrance to Central Park. It had started to rain and we had trouble hailing a taxi to Carnegie Hall. I was late for the ceremony and was still zipping up my soggy gown as the line of students marched down the aisle, but I didn't care. I was so happy to be done. The grandeur of Carnegie Hall, with the gold leaf trim shining from the soaring ceiling, and the luxurious red velvet seats seemed to celebrate with me. Seven years and I was finally done.

I quickly forgot about the VA hospital and Herbert Ziff during the whirlwind of ceremonies, parties, family events, and the framing of my diploma. My grandmother was *kvelling* for the entire weekend. "If only your grandfather Irving could be here," she said with tears. "He'd be so proud of you."

There was a four-week vacation before internship started that July. It was a blissful blur. All I could think about was how happy I was to be done.

∽Five years and an entire residency later I was sitting at a party in the West Village, two blocks from where my NYU graduation had been. Somebody tossed off a flippant comment about medical ethics being just a bunch of "doctor-types and lawyer-types spouting off in the same room." The speaker's words faded as my mind drifted back to my very first ethics meeting as a medical student. I wondered what ever happened to my patient, the first one who'd ever thought of me as his doctor. I was suddenly saddened that I had dropped out of his life and his medical care without ever looking back. A human being's future had been in limbo, but I was too wrapped up in my graduation. I had put him out of sight and out of mind. I couldn't even remember his name. His history had evaporated from my life. Had I passed up an opportunity that would forever be lost?

On a lark, I walked into the medical records office of the VA hospital the following week. I showed them my old student ID card, my finger conveniently covering the expired date, and explained that there was a patient who I had taken care of as a medical student. I didn't remember his last name, only that it started with a Z. But I did know that he had been admitted to the VA shortly before I had graduated medical school. That date I could recite from memory.

The clerk hunted through the computer without success. "I gotta at least know how you spell the last name," she said. "Maybe you got his social security number or date of birth?"

I scoured my memory. "Zall? Zoo? Zink? Zack?" The clerk typed in these variations. Suddenly, Herbert Ziff popped up onto the screen.

The clerk's eyes scanned the screen and I could see her lips moving as she read to herself. Then she reached over and touched my hand. "Honey," she said, "he's been dead two years now."

I lowered my eyes and nodded my head.

The clerk disappeared into a sea of manila charts while I sat in a chipped metal folding chair, fiddling with my outdated ID card. What happens to the charts of dead veterans, I wondered. Did the charts pile up according to rank in some archive in Washington? Was the paper recycled and used to print military manuals? I had almost given up hope, but the U.S. government bureaucracy is apparently indomitable. The clerk reappeared, triumphantly hauling five ungainly folders.

I settled at an unoccupied desk with the stack of charts. Each one was a portly tome with layers upon layers of pages. Where should I begin? Would I ever find the spot where Mr. Ziff and I had crossed paths, where our histories had intersected in that open ward with the long blue curtains? I fingered the edge of the chart. The manila was frayed and softened from the touch of hundreds of thumbs over the years. I placed my own thumb there and slowly opened the cover of the top chart.

I stumbled right upon my own handwriting. I saw the sloppy EKG and my carefully printed admitting orders. I saw my medical student progress notes, all dutifully cosigned by Miguel. Mr. Ziff, zipping around in his wheelchair, sprang back to life. I started reading in earnest from the day of my medical school graduation.

The ethics committee had determined that Mr. Ziff should have the surgery if he could demonstrate his commitment to drug rehab. Six weeks later, he was the proud owner of a spanking new aortic valve. The surgeon's operative note was a half-page long. The only comment was "blood loss limited to 500cc." I marveled at how such terseness could belie the agonizing decision that had preceded the operation.

Mr. Ziff was then transferred to the drug rehab floor. Initially he attended meetings and met with his counselor daily, but then his motivation flagged. One of the nurses' notes quoted Mr. Ziff saying, "I'm only in this rehab because the docs are making me do it." My heart faltered at that and I paused in my reading; I'd been hoping against hope that Mr. Ziff would turn his life around, that he would *want* to turn his life around. All he needed was encouragement and the right environment. I was sure that if I took care of him and went to battle for him and for his valve like a strong, committed doctor should, he would grab the opportunity and begin to live again. I thought I could give him life.

I guess I was naive.

The notes chronicled his increasing disinterest. He began to sleep through group meetings and miss individual appointments. He refused most of his medicines. One month later, a two-line note stated that Mr. Ziff had left AMA—against medical advice. No follow-up visits were recorded.

The next folder documented a brief admission a few months later for alcohol intoxication. There was nothing after that; all the other charts were far older.

I returned the dog-eared manila folders to the clerk and wandered out onto Twenty-third Street. I remembered one time when Mr. Ziff was flying down the hall and screeched his wheelchair to a halt ten feet in front of me. "Doc. Hey Doc," he hollered. "I never seen you wear no skirt before. You got great legs." He turned to one of his hallway cronies. "My doc's got legs." I told him that he had nice legs, too. He grinned and continued wheeling down the hallway to the smoking lounge muttering, "Yeah, my doc's got legs. She got legs . . ."

I wondered about the decision to give him the new valve. Had it been worth it? I leaned against the low brick wall in front of the VA. How could we have given such a patient a new valve? How could we not? I prayed that nobody had gotten stuck with a needle during the operation.

I had no witness to the final two years of Herbert Ziff's life. Did he die in another hospital from repeated infection of his new heart valve? Did he succumb to an AIDS-related illness? Did he get stabbed or shot during a drug deal? Did he end up in prison? Did he freeze to death on the street while passed out from heroin?

I hoped that Mr. Ziff didn't suffer too much pain. I hoped that his wife and daughter had taken care of him toward the end. I hoped that he'd died in his sleep in a warm bed, slumbering gently, dreaming softly, blissfully engaged in his favorite activity.

And I silently thanked him. Mr. Ziff was the first person ever to consider me his doctor. He, more than my diploma or my graduation ceremony, made me feel like a doctor. He helped me over that precipice from medical school to residency. It was still a long climb, but Mr. Ziff boosted me up a few notches. After taking care of him, I was ready to be an intern.

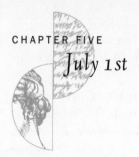

CHAPTER FIVE

July 1st

JULY 1ST. The first day of internship.

Seven years of medical school were finally finished. Graduation in Carnegie Hall was done. Vacation was over. Now I was a real doctor. Of course my grandmother had been referring to me as a doctor for the past seven years, but at least I could stop correcting her now.

I'd decided to stay at Bellevue for internship. I hadn't quite decided if I wanted to pursue internal medicine or neurology. The latter held more opportunities for neuroscience research like I'd done during my Ph.D., but the former seemed more interesting clinically. Since neurology required at least one year of internal medicine training anyway, I figured I'd do a medicine internship and then either switch to neuro or stay on for the full three years of medicine. Staying at Bellevue was the simplest place to do that since the deans and the attendings already knew me and I could probably squeeze in some flexibility. Besides, I'd found a rent-stabilized apartment two blocks away and I would be breaking the cardinal rule of New York City real estate if I gave it up.

I assumed that internship at Bellevue would be just a continuation of medical school, but it wasn't exactly. For starters, all new interns had to be fingerprinted by a New York City police officer. Endless stacks of documents had to be completed. I had to schlep in my framed medical school diploma—photocopies were unacceptable—even though I'd just graduated from the very same institution a few weeks earlier. Among the many forms I had to fill out was one that required my legal signature, copies of which would go to the hospital pharmacy for verifying prescriptions. I hesitated before the long blank line after the words, "Legal Signature of Physician." My official, legal, medical signature.

I grabbed a piece of scrap paper and practiced a few times—after all, I didn't want to put down just any haphazard scribble. Whatever I put down on this line would be the signature that would follow me around for the rest of my professional life. I tried my full name—"Danielle Ofri." Then I experimented with just "D. Ofri." There were time factors to be considered—my first name had eight letters, my last name only four. If I had to sign numerous orders and prescriptions every day as a real doctor, then my first name would slow me down. Maybe I should drop it altogether and just sign "Ofri." It wasn't like there were any other Ofris in Bellevue, or all of Manhattan for that matter. Four letters, short and sweet. And in cursive, once I got past the "O" and the "f," everything else blended into a flourished line, so it was really only two letters. That looked sufficiently succinct and professional. But my driver's license and passport had my full first and last name in the signature. Could there be legal ramifications for having more than one signature? So many new problems to worry about as a doctor.

Then I tagged on an "MD" at the end. How strange looking. Danielle Ofri, MD—that couldn't really be my name residing before those monumental letters, could it? That was the same name I'd trundled along with to nursery school and signed onto my first library card at Finkelstein Memorial Library. How could it possibly have become intimate bedfellows with such austere sounding initials? Then there was the PhD—Danielle Ofri, MD, PhD. No, that was too much. The epithet was now longer than my last name—too portly to be supported by four mere letters. So many possibilities to consider, but I had to take this seriously because my choice now would be my defining professional signature.

After I'd been fingerprinted and documented and verified, I was given a new ID card that said "Housestaff" instead of "Medical Student." I was sure that the new ID card would make me feel like a real doctor. But I felt the same as I had four weeks ago when I was a medical student. In fact, after that month of vacation, I was convinced that I'd forgotten everything I'd known. I couldn't remember Linda's explanation of cardiogenic shock, or Li-Chan's tips on how to draw a blood gas, or Miguel's mnemonic about the causes of metabolic acidosis. And now it was July 1st.

July 1st—that ominous day of beginnings. Once the civilian academic world of high school and college was left behind, the momentous calendar day of beginnings shifted from September to July. Once the world of clinical medicine was entered, September, with its Labor Day gateway, ceased to register any significance on the Gregorian horizon; it was a mere middling month. Even January, with its societally anointed New Year's Day, was just another chit to be passed along. July was now the granite milepost—both threshold and denouement, climax and frontier. July was the yardstick and the chronometer of medicine. Like newly mulched earth at the start of planting season, everything in the medical world was turned over on July 1st. Third-year medical students became fourth-years. Fourth-year students commenced as interns. Interns became residents. Residents reappeared as fellows. Fellows were incarnated as attendings.

July was a month of nervous excitement, each person in the hospital hierarchy kinking their shoulders, adjusting to their new skin. Of course, it was assumed that this process was to be done silently and internally. Outwardly, it was expected that each brick in the pyramid would act as though this unfamiliar identity was a comfortable fit—solid with experience and confidence. On July 1st everyone was expected to walk into their untested roles and act as though they'd been there for years. No one was supposed to admit to the bizarreness of being ratcheted up a notch to a new rank upon the stroke of midnight. One had to comport oneself as though the world of June 30th and prior had never existed, and that July 1st was as smooth as any other day. Or as the interns said, "When in doubt, pretend."

All the new Bellevue interns arrived promptly at 7:15 A.M. on July 1st to receive their list of patients along with a one-time-only free bagel breakfast. All, that is, except me. I had been assigned to begin internship on night-float. Four weeks straight of night shift only.

I spent all day July 1st at home, worrying, while everyone else was at the hospital learning the ropes. At ten o'clock that night I walked through the pitch darkness of First Avenue to Bellevue for my very first day of internship. Eerie yellow lights, as though from an alien spaceship, filtered out from the parking garage next to the hospital. Two old men were leaning against the brick wall drinking out of paper bags. It was too dark to see the Greek columns or garden with the fountain and the birdbath. I walked down the tiny alley under the overhang of the parking garage to the single-door entrance of the Old Bellevue building. The foyer was littered with the day's detritus of coffee cups, candy wrappers, and cigarette butts. Smoke still hung in the air.

I walked alone through the deserted high-arched hallways heading toward New Bellevue, where the real hospital was. The candy shop with its bins of mints and shelves of junk food upon which legions of interns subsisted was closed. The Greek diner that fed the hospital staff who were too disgusted with cafeteria food was closed also, but the lights were still on over the counter. In the mornings there were huge lines snaking out the door—"regular" lanes and "express" lanes. For the uninitiated, it appeared to be utter chaos. Five workers, one with a notably sonorous bass-baritone, would holler back and forth. "Two eggs easy, whiskey down, sesame with a smear, coffee light." Foil-wrapped packages of over-easy eggs, rye toast, and sesame bagel with cream cheese would catapult out of the kitchen, crisscrossing in the air with cups of oatmeal, toasted blueberry muffins, and cinnamon danishes. Filled coffee cups with lids snapped on would sail overhead, only to be snatched out of the air and stuffed into a paper bag without a drop spilled. A fistful of sugars, a couple of grape jellies, and the whole breakfast would be in a bag, ready to go, in less than three minutes. No mix-ups, no errors, no casualties. If only the laboratory staff was as efficient as the coffee shop guys, the interns often moaned.

Old Bellevue now housed only administrative offices—all the patients had been moved to New Bellevue in the 1970s. But I remembered

Dr. Weiser, an older gynecology professor, telling us about his residency in the Old Bellevue building. Young women would flood the emergency room, he told us, hemorrhaging from back-alley abortions. The interns would load them onto stretchers and haul them up the stairs to the operating rooms. There were no elevators or transport orderlies. Up and down the steps the interns lugged their human cargo. A race to control the bleeding. Even now I could see the dips worn into the stone steps by generations of Bellevue interns carrying their patients. I wondered if I could have balanced a stretcher while climbing those steep stairs. And what could it have felt like to be a frightened, bleeding patient jostling up the bumpy incline, watching the molded ceiling jerk overhead like a disjointed filmstrip? "You kids don't know what it was like back then," Dr. Weiser had said quietly, shaking his head. "You're not old enough to remember those days. But I do. They bled to death before we even got them up the stairs. Or died of overwhelming infection." He paused and sighed. "You kids just don't know."

On the second floor of Old Bellevue, just down from the Benefits office, was Chapel Hall. Sixteen-foot ceilings and arched doorways led to this little-used corner of Bellevue. There were three chapels side by side—Catholic, Protestant, and Jewish. Stained glass, dark oak paneling, corniced molding, delicately fluted windows, glowing candles. Each room was a spacious, peaceful sanctuary. The wooden doors were always open, inviting. I never actually saw anybody inside, but the stately pews and dark, bound books looked well tended and freshly arranged. There might have been religious services for patients, or perhaps employees drifted in for private meditation, but I never witnessed the rooms being used. Whenever I passed by them on my way to submit another dull pile of forms regarding my latest dental claim to the Benefits office, I would peek into these quiet cavernous houses of worship, these hidden jewels of Bellevue. Such generous rooms would never be apportioned in a modern building. These, like the fountain and birdbath in the garden, were truly relics of the nineteenth century. I felt that here was where the ghosts of Bellevue resided. Ghosts of interns past who sprinted up those stone stairs literally carrying their patients in their arms. Ghosts of patients whose lives began in so many corners of the world, but ground to a halt in this brick building. Occasionally I'd duck into the Jewish chapel for a few minutes of solitude in my otherwise chaotic days. The wooden ark waited patiently, quietly dignified, ready to receive multitudes or just me. The silver menorah was polished, reflecting whoever was there or had been there. I felt the reassuring presence of those ghosts; I was never alone.

I turned the corner where Old Bellevue connected with the New Bellevue building. Suddenly the curved plaster moldings gave way to steel and glass. The quirky angles and unpredictable crannies dissolved into rigid parallel lines and twentieth-century utilitarian geometry. Luckily—perhaps in deference to the architects of Old Bellevue—the creators of New Bellevue were not too stingy with space, and the halls and rooms of the new hospital were relatively airy. There was no fancy architecture in New Bellevue, but I did appreciate the modern elevators. Since the stairwells were locked, the elevators were a necessity and like the morning lines in the coffee shop, they came in "local" and "express" varieties.

The waiting area by the elevators was deserted at this time of night. The security guard slurped her coffee and barely glanced up from her magazine to check my ID. My brand new ID. The one that now said "MD" after my name. She didn't even notice.

I shuffled in place. My new white coat was clean and pressed, and the insignia said "NYU Medical Center," instead of "NYU School of Medicine." Subtle distinction, perhaps, to the world beyond First Avenue and Twenty-seventh Street, but portentous inside these hallways. Being part of the medical *center* instead of the medical *school* meant that I had finally expanded beyond the self-indulgent chrysalis of studenthood, in which the overriding purpose of illness, trauma, and patients had been the absorption of knowledge. Yes, I'd comforted myself back then with the fact that this knowledge was being acquired for the betterment of my future patients, but still I was nagged by the self-centered inequity of it. But now, sporting the insignia of the medical center I was officially part of the housestaff—one of the interns that made Bellevue run. Of course, I was still learning, but the primary reason for my existence on the hospital floor was now to take care of patients, not myself. I no longer had to justify my presence next to a suffering human being; I had a purpose. My new ID and new insignia confirmed that. I smoothed my coat, even though it had only the large creases from the industrial pressing machine in the laundry department.

A group of loud-talking surgeons sauntered out of the elevator, sporting ratty scrubs under their stained white coats. I entered the empty elevator in their wake, conscious of the silence and the neatly pressed white coat that hung around me. But our coats, worn or new, all shared the same insignia. I was finally part of the team.

The sixteenth floor "on-call" room was our headquarters. If it had been cleaned for July 1st, it wasn't apparent to me. Interns and residents were flopped on the tattered blue couches, exhausted after their first day on call. White coats, IVs, syringes, and pink progress notes were strewn about the tables and couches. An X-ray folder—white with red trim—lay on the floor. A footprint was smudged on it, and four black films spilled out. The TV was tuned to a late-night comedy show. At the center table was a night-float resident who looked to be in charge. A bountiful supply of potato chips, soda, chocolate bars, and pretzels was laid out before him. A forlorn bag of carrot sticks sat at the end next to a puddle of coffee that had spilled and long since solidified.

"You a night-float intern?" he called out to me. He was leaning back in his chair, aiming plastic forks javelin-style into the garbage pail with remarkable accuracy. I nodded and moved toward the table. "Name's Kevin," he said, sinking another fork into the pail then nodding with satisfaction. Kevin was long and lean, with three days of beard growth smudging his cheeks. "Property of Boston City Hospital" was emblazoned in spotty black print in random places on his green scrubs, reminding me of an overseas package with "Air Mail" stamped on every available spot by an overeager postal worker. "Get your sign-out sheets from the interns so they can go home, then we'll have some breakfast. The pretzels are fresh this morning."

The on-call intern waved a fistful of sign-out sheets at me—his and those of the other three interns he'd been covering. Each sheet contained the barely legible, scrawled summary of ten patients. A brief history of each patient, along with the medications, IVs, allergies, DNR status, and fever threshold were compressed into one-inch rows. When a patient was discharged, the intern would "erase" that patient by affixing a line of one-inch white labels across the row that had contained that patient's information. The new patient's information would be scrawled in the new blank row. Of course the labels were not entirely opaque so some of the previous patient's information always shone through. Eventually the sign-out sheets became stiff like cardboard with layer upon layer of scribbled-upon white labels. The sheets, now more akin to multimedia modern artworks, no longer folded like normal paper, but cracked at the crease lines, at which point surgical tape was used to fasten the loose pieces together. In these days, before computers were readily available to provide daily updated, pristine printouts, interns prided themselves in making it through an entire month rotation without ever having to rewrite their sign-outs.

The on-call intern shoved a stack of thick, cracked papers at me in one crumpled bunch. "Nothing much happening," he said. "Just check if Mrs. Sing's potassium's back. And Escalera on 17-West died about two hours ago. I took care of the paperwork and everything, but his family might call." He plunked the stiff sheets of illegible hieroglyphics in my hands, grabbed his coat, and started out the door. "Oh, the nurses called me about some lady who fell out of bed on 16-East. But it was already ten o'clock, so I told them that you'd take care of it." The door slammed and he was gone.

Night-float was supposed to be the direct continuation of medical care from the day teams. But since I had the patient load of four interns, this was impossible. I couldn't get to know forty patients—there just wasn't time between the hundreds of little tasks I was being paged to do.

My beeper never stopped. "Mr. Rivera on 19-South needs a new IV." "Ms. Ahmed on 16-West has a fever." "Mr. Soto in the CCU is having chest pain." "Can we get an order for restraints for Ms. Sherry on 17-

West?" "Mr. Rivera's IV is out again." "Mrs. Quan on 15-West is refusing her meds." "Mr. Helal's daughter is here and wants to speak to a doctor." "Mrs. Noland on 16-East is having a reaction to her blood transfusion." "Dr. Rashid wrote an order this morning for antibiotics, but it conflicts with Dr. Levy's order. Can you come figure it out?" "Mr. Rivera's IV is out *again!*" Night-float turned out to be damage control—getting the patients through the night until the interns returned in the morning.

I raced from one ward to the next, patching this problem, calming that one, counting the hours until the day interns would return. But my technical skills improved rapidly because there was so much to do and no one else to do it for me. Within a few days I was able to draw double sets of blood cultures in semidarkness. I could do a blood gas on the first try. I found that I only had to call Kevin for the really difficult IVs in the drug users who had no veins.

Kevin was the model laid-back resident, comfortably unshaven and insouciantly grungy. The cares of the everyday world didn't seem to faze him. That impressed me to no end. I always worried about getting enough sleep, about finding something decent to eat, about getting all my work done, about fitting all the paraphernalia I'd need in my pockets, about getting called for something I couldn't handle. Kevin seemed to be perpetually relaxed. All through the night as I returned from this or that task, I'd find him in the call room with his feet up on the table, his hand on the remote control, the *New York Times* and a bag of chips opened at his side. Yet, at eight A.M., when the day teams would arrive, there'd be a stack of at least three or four admissions that he'd worked up during the night, with thoroughly written histories neatly tucked inside the red-and-white X-ray folder for each patient. The pockets of his white coat were nearly empty of stuff, yet the times I saw him at a patient's bedside, he always managed to pull the exact needed piece of equipment from his pocket.

Kevin's vocabulary was comfortably sprinkled with scatological references to the patients he admitted. On good days he merely referred to the patients from the nursing homes as gomes. The term gomer came from a popular medical novel, *The House of God,* and was originally an acronym for "Get Out Of My Emergency Room," but it had taken on a life of its own. Gomes, or gomers, now meant any demented or homeless patient who was undesirable. Gome-docs were meagerly trained doctors out in the community who sent half-dead patients to the hospital for useless evaluations.

With his slow drawl, Kevin railed against the gome-docs as he flipped the channels from B-movie to off-hour cooking show to late-night comedy. In a roundabout way I was reassured that with this residency training, I would be protected from ever turning into a gomedoc.

I was always a little nervous calling Kevin for help, but he'd answer promptly in an amiably grumpy voice. Usually he'd try to walk me through the problem over the phone, but if I was really stuck, he'd saunter over to whichever ward I was stranded on with his hands crammed into the pockets of his white coat and help me interpret an EKG or talk down an agitated patient.

Life at night started taking on its own comforting routine. I'd show up at ten P.M. in my most comfortable old clothes. I'd get my signouts and then settle in for a good junk-food breakfast with Kevin and the other night-floaters. Then I would make "Tylenol rounds" to all the nursing stations—writing, in advance, all the Tylenol orders that I'd inevitably be paged for in the middle of the night. I'd try to be proactive, tying up as many loose ends as possible to spare myself being paged later on. And then I'd begin my journey from one brush fire to the next, keeping the chaos under moderate control until the day interns returned. I discovered that the south staircase was unlocked between the sixteenth and seventeenth floors, so I didn't have to rely on the elevators. My calves got plenty of exercise.

I grew accustomed to trudging out of the hospital at nine A.M., fighting the incoming traffic of freshly showered and coifed employees. I trained myself to sleep through the bright, sunny summer days. Day sleep, I learned, was never as thorough as night sleep, and never long enough. But it was, in some ways, more efficient. Upon plopping into bed at 9:30 A.M., I would plunge directly into Stage IV sleep, skipping all the other preliminary stages. I'd wake up a few hours later, grab some food, then drop right back into Stage IV sleep. And there was always an overtone of mischevious delight in day sleep. Sleeping during the day I'd always associated with playing hooky or taking a siesta while on vacation. And while I knew that I'd just completed a full "day's" work and had earned this sleep, I felt an extra twinge of smug satisfaction that I'd somehow beaten the system, that I was snuggling into bed while the rest of New York City was facing a whole depressing day of work in their cubicles or assembly lines. I purposely did not close the blinds on my windows. I wanted to experience every bit of sunlight to make my sleep feel the most sneakily delicious. I would turn on my bedside radio to the morning newscast as I settled under my covers. And I would sail off to Stage IV sleep, blithely ignoring the world events and traffic reports on my radio that the rest of the world was forced to contend with.

One night during my third week of night-float, Kevin paged me at three A.M. "Elba Rodriguez's blood count just dropped 13 points," he said. "Get over to 16-North and figure out where she's bleeding from."

I raced down the stairs and ran into Kevin walking out of Mrs. Rodriguez's room. "I just took her blood pressure and did a repeat blood count," he said. "Go do a rectal exam and see if she's bleeding from her GI tract." My pocket was already stocked with gloves, petroleum jelly, and test cards to check for blood in the stool. I strode into the room—crack night-float intern—ready for battle.

Mrs. Rodriguez was a tiny, wrinkled Dominican woman with frizzy gray hair amassed on the pillow. She was wearing a worn, floral housecoat and cardigan sweater over her hospital gown. Her daughter, grandson, and a few other relatives stood gathered around her bed. They all turned and looked at me with concern on their faces.

I cleared my throat. "Hi, I'm Dr. Ofri." I hoped that sounded convincing. "I'm one of the night doctors taking care of Mrs. Rodriguez. I know the other doctor was already here to see her. I'm just here to do the rectal exam." Yep, Dr. Ofri, rectal specialist!

The grandson stepped forward. He was slim and amber-skinned. A small moustache graced his upper lip. "I understand what you have to do. I'm a nurse. If you don't mind, I'd like to stay here while you do it."

My grip on the metal railing of the bed tightened. Stay while I do the rectal?

"Well, I ... um ..." Were family members allowed to be present for rectals? But he was a nurse. "I ... if you ... well ..." Where was Kevin? Why wasn't I home in bed like the rest of the civilized world?

I gestured somewhat inanely in the air and shrugged my shoulders. "Whatever you want, I guess."

The rest of the family left the room. I pulled the curtain so that Mrs. Rodriguez, the grandson, and I were separated from the three other sleeping patients. The grandson stood to Mrs. Rodriguez's right, and I stood to her left. We rolled her toward the grandson, and I fumbled with her housecoat, cardigan sweater, and hospital gown to get down to her skin. I fished around in my pockets to unearth the necessary equipment and suddenly realized that I was missing the little bottle of developer fluid to do the test for blood in the stool.

I looked over to the grandson, who was balancing his grandmother on her right side. "Umm, could you hold her there for just one minute? I need to get one more thing." I dashed out of the room, studiously avoiding eye contact with the family members waiting in the hall.

I ran into the 16-North supply closet but there wasn't any developer fluid on the shelf. I dug through the drawers and the storage bins but I couldn't find any; all the other interns had probably pocketed them. I raced out of the supply closet, down the hall, around the corner to 16-West. I tore through the supplies in their closet, sweating under my polyester coat. No developer fluid.

The cardiac care unit! They were always well stocked. I knew the nurses guarded their supplies like hawks, so I snuck into the CCU from the back door where the bedpans and dirty laundry were kept. I tip-toed over to the supply shelf in the far corner: IVs, chest tubes, iodine swabs, glycerin swabs. Where was the damn developer fluid? Aha! Tucked behind the 5cc syringes was a yellow bottle of developer. I snatched it just as a nurse yelled, "Hey, those are CCU supplies." I jammed the bottle in my pocket and dashed out of the CCU with my head down. From the back all interns looked alike, I hoped.

I was panting when I got back to Mrs. Rodriguez's room. Her grandson was still balancing her on her right side. His face was calm, and he didn't say a word.

I gloved up and slathered my right index finger with petroleum jelly. Gingerly I slid my finger into Mrs. Rodriguez's rectum. I bit my lower lip as I concentrated on my assigned task. I felt around, hunting for any abnormal masses. I wriggled my finger attempting to snag a sample of stool to check for blood. Rectal tone, I reminded myself. Don't forget to assess for adequate rectal tone.

Good job, I complimented myself, as my fingertip hooked onto a suitably firm piece of stool. I'll just pull out this little tidbit, smear it on the card, plop some developer fluid on it and maybe I'll be able to get some sleep before the nurses do their six A.M. vitals and start calling me with the next round of fevers.

"I think Mamy is no longer with us," the grandson quietly announced.

I froze in mid-rectal and looked up at the grandson. His calm expression hadn't changed. My heart began to pound inside my ears. No longer with us? What was he talking about?

With his free hand, the grandson crossed himself thoughtfully and murmured something in Spanish.

No longer with us? Mrs. Rodriguez was dead? The bit of stool was still hooked onto my fingertip. I could feel a hot stickiness tingling under my shirt.

How could she be dead?

The grandson let out a soft sigh. "Mamy didn't want any extraordinary measures. We signed the DNR together. I'm so glad we didn't do any machines or tubes. It's the way she wanted it—drifting off in peace. We just need you to pronounce her dead, Doctor, then we can take her home."

I stared at the grandson, blinking repetively as my mind blanked out to nothingness. The window beyond him was pitch-black. There was no moon. A few faint lights twinkled from across the river. I couldn't remember where I was or what I was doing here. I could only hear my heart thud rythmically.

Dead! That's right, Mrs. Rodriguez is dead! My own breathing resumed, and I realized that I should probably remove my index finger from Mrs. Rodriguez's rectum. I slid my hand out and stared at it blankly. Dead ... Mrs. Rodriguez is dead.

I tore the glove off. Suddenly my mind began to race—how do I declare a patient dead?

Pupillary reflexes. That's it. A dead person doesn't have pupillary reflexes. I pulled out my flashlight and shone it confidently in Mrs. Rodriguez's eyes. To my dismay, she had huge cataracts; she wouldn't have pupillary reflexes anyway.

Respirations. A dead person won't breathe. I whipped out my stethoscope. By now the whole family had come in from the hallway and gathered around the bedside. They followed my every move as I inserted the stethoscope in my ears and carefully planted the bell on Mrs. Rodriguez's chest. I listened carefully. Suddenly a vibrating twitch ran through her body. I jumped back and the family looked at me with worried eyes. Was this rigor mortis, or might she still be alive? It suddenly dawned on me that I'd never had a lecture in medical school on how to tell if someone is dead. I guess it was assumed to be pretty obvious—dead is dead, and if you're not dead then you're alive, right? I thought about paging Kevin, but the family was staring intently at me. How could I leave now?

Pulse, that's it. Dead people for sure don't have a pulse. I ran my fingers along her left carotid. And then along her right carotid. Of course, the only way you know you've found the pulse is when you find the pulse. How do you know when you haven't found one? How do you document the absence of something when its presence is defined by hunting until you've found it? Maybe I just wasn't feeling in the right place. I fumbled through her folds of skin and neck muscles. Maybe the pulse was hidden behind the sternocleidomastiod muscle.

It wasn't there. Did that mean she was dead or that I just couldn't find it? Maybe it was a half-inch to the right. Maybe it was deeper, or maybe I was pressing too hard. Was I supposed to cover every inch of her body to prove that I couldn't find a pulse?

Another shiver ran through her body and then echoed through mine.

The family looked at me, their eyes gathered in a single longing stare, waiting for an answer. How could I say anything? What if I got it wrong?

An EKG. That's it. If I get a flat line on the EKG then I'll have proof that she's dead. Nobody could argue with a flat line. I excused myself and dashed back to the supply closet to get the EKG machine. I wheeled the dilapidated machine to Mrs. Rodriguez's bedside. The ten leads were hopelessly knotted. I struggled with the tangled cords, twisting and pulling, muttering curses under my breath at whichever intern had used the machine last.

There were four rubber wristbands for her wrists and ankles. I looped them around, trying to catch the metal hooks into the holes in the rubber, but they sloshed recklessly amidst the overgenerous supply of electrode jelly I'd applied.

The six chest leads sported red rubber suctions cups. I pinched each one to get sufficient suction to stick them onto Mrs. Rodriguez's chest. As I squeezed them, ancient electrode jelly from EKGs gone by slithered out in crusted blue clumps. Mrs. Rodriguez didn't have much bulk for the suction cups to grab onto; as soon as I fastened one onto her chest, the previous one I'd placed would pop off. I applied more jelly and then re-squeezed the suction cups. Pop! Another one flew off. The grandson and family bent in closer and followed with their eyes back and forth as I chased down the obstreperous suction cups. The more jelly I applied, the more they popped off. I wiped away the hair that had fallen in my face and a slimy gob of electrode jelly slid down my forehead. The stiff polyester collar of my white coat was plastered to my neck, cutting off all air supply to my body.

Finally the EKG was completely set up. I sucked in my cheeks and hit the start button. We all stared at the skinny strip of graph paper snaking out from the machine. Please, I prayed, be a flat line—something I could hang on to.

The paper emerged with unreadable squiggles. Between the air vents and the three IV pumps running in the next bed over, there was too much background noise. I jiggled around the EKG leads, but I could not get a stable baseline. Two more suction cups popped off.

The grandson curled his hand around his grandmother's wrist. "She's dead, Doctor," he said softly. "She has no pulse. You don't have to do any more tests."

My face was burning and I could only stare at the EKG electrodes that continued to pop off her chest.

The grandson continued. "Mamy lived a long and wonderful life, but now she's dead. We are grateful that we could at least be with her at her last moments." The family joined hands and began to recite a prayer in Spanish.

The weight of my white coat, laden with its instruments of medicine, pulled at my neck; the stiff material chafed against my clammy skin. I stood in silence while they prayed, coaxing moisture from my throat to wet my parched mouth. As their lips mumbled in unison, I tried to imagine the cool peacefulness of the chapels in the Old Bellevue building—the soothing marble and comforting oak panels. The stripe of electrode jelly on my forehead had solidified. My shirt was damp with sweat. Five feet of EKG strips was crumpled in my sticky palm.

When they were done I unhooked all the EKG leads. I wiped the blobs of blue jelly from Mrs. Rodriguez's chest and closed her gown. I helped the grandson replace her housecoat and cardigan sweater. I grabbed the EKG machine and started backing it and myself out of the room. "I, um, I'm sorry," I whispered hoarsely. "About your grandmother, that is. And if you, uh, need anything . . . don't hesitate . . ." The back wheels of the machine abruptly swerved left and I collided with the doorframe. "Anything . . . really."

I jerked the EKG machine out of the room and collapsed into a chair in the nurses' station. My face was rippling with heat and embarrassment. How could I not figure out whether or not Mrs. Rodriguez was dead? Wasn't that what doctors did—pronounce the time of death? How could I ever be a doctor if I couldn't tell a dead person from a live one? I had my diploma tucked away in my apartment; I had those extra "MD" letters after my name; I had the medical center insignia on my white coat—and I couldn't distinguish life from death? When were all these magical medical skills supposed to materialize?

I slumped over in my chair. The mountain before me seemed impossibly steep. I thought I'd already climbed so high, what with four years of college and seven years of medical school. I'd already passed the first two parts of the medical boards. But it seemed that I was at the beginning again, craning my neck upward toward an insurmountable slope of knowledge. How could there exist so much to be ignorant of? Hadn't I made any progress in the last eleven years? I brushed the hair out of my face and blue electrode jelly snagged under my fingernails. What was I going to write on the death certificate as the immediate cause of death . . . rectal exam?

Kevin materialized in the nurses' station, without me even having to call him. He helped me sort through Mrs. Rodriguez's chart and fill out the death certificate. We listed Alzheimer's disease as the cause of death at age ninety, and Kevin didn't use the word gome once. I wrote a brief "expiration note" in the chart. I didn't mention the rectal exam.

In the morning I staggered home in the brilliant July sun. A hot shower washed away the last of the electrode jelly. A cup of tea and warm toast eased some of the aches. The crisp summer colors—azure cloudless sky, green trees sharply outlined between brownstones, brilliantly reflective glass skyscrapers—soothed my eyes and chased away the endless darkness of night-float duty. I crawled into bed, grateful for the soft, clean cotton sheets. I drifted off to sleep, thinking of Elba Rodriguez. I imagined her as a young woman, a fresh immigrant to America with her three children. I thought of her ninety years of life, of growing old in her Brooklyn neighborhood. I imagined that she'd been a regular patient at the Bellevue clinic all her life, coming every year to the old brick building for her annual physical. Maybe she'd given birth to her children at Bellevue. Maybe she'd prayed on occasion in the chapel. Maybe she expected that she would die at Bellevue. Perhaps her spirit had already joined the other ghosts in the chapel. I hoped that wherever she was now, she forgave me for the indignities she suffered at the hands of an inexperienced intern.

"I'll do better next time, Mrs. Rodriguez," I whispered aloud as I drifted off to sleep, the morning traffic report bleating from the radio. "For the next patient, I'll do better. Just give me some time."

CHAPTER SIX

The Professor of Denial

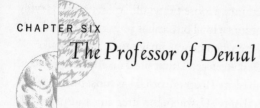

WE HAD JUST FINISHED taking the history from the patient when Lee, the medical student, piped in. He had just started on the wards and was eager to practice his interviewing skills. "And what do you think is causing your illness?" he asked earnestly. I remembered being taught that same technique when I was a third-year student.

Dr. Schwartz turned toward Lee. "Viral hepatitis," he clipped. "I've got every classic sign. Go back and read your *Harrison's*." With that he snatched the November issue of *Archives of Psychiatry* from his bed-side and started flipping through the pages. I shifted my weight and lowered my eyes to the ground. Sandy, my resident, pursed her lips and a small sigh came out. Only Lee appeared unfazed.

Loose bags of skin hung off Dr. Schwartz's spindly bones, and his eyes were sucked into his skull. Any muscle he'd once possessed had long since withered. The chart said he was sixty-seven years old but he looked eighty. When we'd asked, he'd said he had only been sick for a week or two.

His belt had four extra holes punched in to gather in the expansive pleats of his pants, but he denied losing any weight. His skin, eyes, and tongue emitted an eerie yellow glow that seemed almost artificial. His liver was the size of a football and brick-hard.

Viral hepatitis? I'd seen spunkier-looking cadavers in anatomy lab.

Sandy, Lee, and I withdrew into the hallway and his wife followed us out. "He's been sick for more than a year," Mrs. Schwartz confided, her long, graying hair tucked into a loose ponytail. "We have been trying to get him to see a doctor for so long but he has refused. We could only bring him into the hospital when he was finally too weak to walk."

Just two blocks up First Avenue, University Hospital was a world away from Bellevue. University Hospital, or UH as most people called it, was the private hospital of NYU, where the attendings admitted patients from their private practices. As a private hospital, UH was privy to all of the latest amenities that money could buy.

UH, however, was torture for us interns. Every patient had a private attending and a panoply of specialists to make all the interesting medical decisions. The interns were rarely included in these discussions. We spent our days drawing blood, renewing medication orders, writing notes in the chart that nobody ever read, fetching test results, doing EKGs, and replacing IVs in the middle of the night. When we entered patients' rooms, they scrutinized our ID cards to weed out the housestaff, preferring to wait for their "real" doctors.

To a Bellevue patient, anybody in a white coat was a doctor.

Internship was divided into one-month rotations. The bulk of our rotations were spent on the Bellevue medical wards. One month was on the UH wards. Another month was night float. One month each was spent in the Bellevue and UH intensive care units. Any time at UH was dreaded. Although it was fun seeing all the high-tech gadgets, we were on call every third night instead of every fourth as at Bellevue (on the absurd premise that because the patients had private doctors, there was less work for us to do). UH patients, by virtue of having better outpatient care than Bellevue patients, were much older and sicker by the time they were admitted to the hospital, and therefore much more work for the interns. There were no homeless patients languishing on the wards awaiting a bed at the shelter. There were no undocumented aliens waiting around for Medicaid. Every patient at UH was actively sick, usually with three or four major illnesses. There was certainly a lot of medicine to learn at UH, but staying afloat in the sea of scut with forty attendings breathing down your back left most interns too exhausted to muster any spare neurons for education.

. . .

&I learned from Mrs. Schwartz that her husband was a bigwig in the Freudian psychoanalytic world. He had published extensively and ran a busy clinical practice for decades. He had continued to practice until just recently, when his increasing fatigue forced him to slow his pace. He was also a travel buff. They had toured all through India and China as well as South America. They'd been on a Caribbean cruise only two months ago.

A CT scan of his abdomen showed an enlarged liver and gallbladder with massively dilated bile ducts leading out of the liver, suggesting a mass obstructing the outflow. The radiologist turned to me and shook his head. "The top three diagnoses are pancreatic cancer, pancreatic cancer, and pancreatic cancer."

That's it, I thought as I left the radiology suite, the game is over. A diagnosis of pancreatic cancer is essentially a death sentence. It's not that the cancer per se is so malevolent, but its hallmark is that it is only detected after malignant spread to other abdominal organs. If, by chance, it is caught before metastasizing, it is theoretically curable by surgical removal, but that is rarely the case. Usually patients enter the hospital, get their diagnosis of pancreatic cancer, then die shortly afterward. Life expectancy is generally a matter of weeks to months; precipitous decline could occur at any moment.

Dr. Gursky was the attending on the case. He was a short, trim man with a bustling private practice in the hospital's faculty practice building. He rounded on his hospitalized patients before 6:00 in the morning, then did evening rounds at about eight P.M. We rarely saw him during the day, and his notes in the chart consisted of one or two succinct lines of inscrutable text. Since this was UH, and not Bellevue, we were obliged to carry out his orders, but it was a challenge to decipher them. We didn't want to call him every day about every single patient, and it was difficult to reach him by phone, anyway, because he was so busy at his office. We often resorted to asking the patients what he'd told them about their plan for the day, but they'd usually been sound asleep when Dr. Gursky made his predawn rounds. And so the guessing game would continue all day as we'd ask each other to take a stab at interpreting one hieroglyphic note or another. If we saw him in the hall, we'd rush to ask all of our accumulated questions. I ran into Dr. Gursky later that week in the hospital cafeteria. I asked him if he had brought up the issues of DNR and hospice care with Dr. Schwartz and his family. "Well," he replied, filling his paper cup with coffee, "we can't be one hundred percent sure that it is pancreatic cancer until we do a biopsy. It could very well be intestinal cancer or bile duct cancer." He poured in a splash of milk. "I don't want to lay out all those issues until we're absolutely sure of the diagnosis and prognosis. It wouldn't be fair to the patient." He looked down at his watch. "Sorry, gotta run. I'll catch you guys tomorrow." He stuffed two packets of sugar in his pocket and strode out the door.

The prognosis and treatment options, of course, could not be fully explored until an oncologist had consulted on the case. The oncologist would not see the patient until a biopsy was done. The biopsy would only be obtained after the gastroenterologist had consulted on the patient. The surgeon would not evaluate the patient for possible removal of the mass until the gastroenterologist had performed the biopsy, the pathologist had evaluated the biopsy, and the oncologist had reviewed the results. Did Dr. Schwartz have enough time for all these specialists?

I reluctantly agreed that Dr. Gursky had a point about diagnostic certainty, but given Dr. Schwartz's emaciated state, I couldn't imagine that it could possibly alter the outcome. His only hope for a cure was surgical removal, but the tumor, whatever type it was, was hopelessly tangled in a knot of veins, arteries, and bile ducts. And even if surgery were technically feasible, the operation itself could kill him. Weakened, malnourished patients were always more prone to the complications of anesthesia and post-op infections. To me, the potential complications seemed numerous and the benefits dubious.

As an intern at UH my opinion was about as valuable as that of the janitor. My job was to make sure that the IVs were in and the blood was drawn every day.

Thus, the quest for a "tissue diagnosis" went forth. Dr. Schwartz initially refused the biopsy. Mrs. Schwartz pleaded with him to find out exactly what diagnosis he had. Dr. Gursky lectured him about diagnostic algorithms. Throughout much of this haranguing, Dr. Schwartz kept his nose buried in medical journals, raising his head only to say that he was not interested, thank you very much, and that the viral hepatitis would resolve on its own.

Finally, after days of begging and cajoling, he consented. "Just to get you all to leave me alone so I can get some work done," he'd said, flipping the pages of the *American Journal of Psychiatry*. "I need some peace and quiet to work."

The next day a gastroenterologist passed a tube from Dr. Schwartz's mouth through his stomach to his intestine. A tiny probe explored his pancreas and procured a biopsy. Another tortuous week of IVs and blood draws elapsed while the pathologists preserved, sliced, stained, and examined the specimens. The final result was "nonspecific changes, nondiagnostic tissue specimen." The whole exercise had to be repeated.

Dr. Schwartz was cantankerous but he had a soft spot for the house-staff. He hated the needles, but tolerated the many sticks that I gave him. "You should've seen me as an intern," he boasted in his gravelly voice as I stuck him for the third time that morning. "I was the handiest one with a needle. Whenever there was a tough IV, they'd come get me. I almost went for a surgical residency. I considered it seriously for quite some time, but psychoanalysis was the place for intellectuals—the place for real thinkers."

On morning rounds, Dr. Schwartz offered us psychological profiles of the staff. "You know that cleaning woman? The one with the red hair? She has control issues. Watch her when she comes in, you'll see. She stakes out her space with the mop and doesn't let anyone invade. Not even the nurses. The whole ward is held up till she's done."

Then he would launch into a tirade against whatever procedure was planned for that day. "You people just want to torture me. You want to stick a tube into every hole I've got. I just have a touch of hepatitis; it'll get better on its own. Get away from me already, I've got a lot of important reading to do."

"Abe, it's just one more test," Mrs. Schwartz pleaded. Her hair was slipping out from its ponytail. "We've got to find out what's making you feel sick." She took his hand and placed it in her lap. His fingers looked even yellower against her pale blue slacks. She traced her finger along one of his. "Please, Abe."

Dr. Schwartz grimaced and snorted, staring out the window. He withdrew his hand and grabbed another journal from the nightstand. He stared at the cover and then tossed it back on to the pile. "Okay. But just this one test. That's it." And another tube would be stuck into another hole.

Over the next week or two, he began to refuse his tests more vehemently. He would close his eyes and rebuff any attempts to reason with him. "Leave me alone, you people," was his daily retort. "Can't a body get some rest around here?" He even refused the nurses' assistance with bathing. A wild scruffy white beard overtook his gaunt face.

The tube that had been placed in his liver drained the yellow bilirubin from his skin. In its wake was left another chemical, biliverdin, which lent a greenish hue to his increasingly macabre appearance.

Dr. Schwartz showed less and less interest in food. He pushed his meal trays away without even opening them. "This is pitiful," he said. "This whole place is pitiful." He stopped sitting up in bed and the current issue of *Psychoanalytic Quarterly* sat on his nightstand unopened. He just lay in his bed and barked at anyone who got too close.

Every meal, every blood test, every IV, became an ordeal. The staff dreaded going into his room. When it became clear that his nutritional status was swiftly sinking, a feeding tube was placed through his nose into his stomach. Dr. Schwartz was not interested in our exhortations about his need to gain strength and the importance of nutrition for his immune system. He simply yanked it out as soon as the nurse left the room.

Each time he pulled it out, the trusty intern was called upon to replace it. Dr. Schwartz fought me desperately as I tried to cram the plastic tube in his nose. He spat and clawed as I forced it down his throat. Dr. Gursky ordered mittens and restraints for his hands. The tube still managed to come out every night. Tied down, Dr. Schwartz's body would convulse with rage as I gritted my teeth and forced the tube in over and over again. I pleaded with him to stop fighting, to stop making our torture session any worse than it had to be. I felt like I was being forced to rape him.

But interns didn't make decisions at UH. If Dr. Schwartz were at Bellevue, I'd have let him stay without the feeding tube. If he was going to die in several weeks what did it matter if he had a few more or a few less carbohydrates? If he only had a little time left on earth, why should he be tortured with this damn plastic tube? Why should I?

After the tube-feeding debacle, a central line was placed in a large neck vein for artificial nutrition. This too he managed to dislodge, placing him at risk for dangerous air bubbles in his vein. Extra restraints were added.

Meanwhile the endoscopy had been repeated and the biopsy was again nondiagnostic. Dr. Gursky was talking with the surgeons about taking Dr. Schwartz to the operating room to get a definitive biopsy and attempt resection if feasible.

Mrs. Schwartz visited every day, even though her husband was barely communicative and increasingly contemptuous of her. She sat silently next to his bed, knitting or reading, while he stared out the window, his journals and books untouched on the nightstand. She was making a pink scarf for her grandniece, who was turning eight next month. Sometimes Mrs. Schwartz gave up and just stared out the window also. There was almost no conversation in that room.

Whenever I could catch Dr. Gursky in the hallway, I would ask him about broaching the DNR issue. Theoretically, do not resuscitate orders were supposed to be discussed with every patient upon admission to the hospital, but I rarely saw it happen. Without a DNR order, any patient who stopped breathing or whose heart stopped beating would be subject to resuscitation, or, in hospital lingo, a code. A code consisted of cardiopulmonary resuscitation (CPR) with compressions on the chest, and intubation with a breathing tube, as well as powerful intravenous medications to help jumpstart the heart. A DNR allowed a patient to forego this. For anyone with a terminal disease, a DNR seemed like a good idea to me. Why should they be subjected to such torture when their disease was going to kill them anyway?

At this point Dr. Schwartz clearly did not have decisional capacity for such weighty issues. The burden would now fall on his wife. I was frustrated because I felt we had missed the window of opportunity for Dr. Schwartz to articulate his thoughts and feelings. Did he want a DNR? How much more medical testing did he want? What exactly would he want us to do if he stopped breathing? Would he want a breathing machine? Dr. Gursky agreed in principle, but felt that it would be unfair to make any predictions without a tissue diagnosis.

I felt like a collaborator in Dr. Schwartz's indignities: I was the one who had to sign the daily orders for him to be tied down—"for patient safety." He was now wearing a diaper because he wouldn't, and now couldn't, get out of bed to use the commode. Even more distressing was that he ceased to protest in his old cantankerous manner. Now he just grunted and turned his head away. He was too restrained to roll over.

Mrs. Schwartz absorbed this metamorphosis silently. Her outspoken, opinionated husband had been transformed into a babbling infant. The man she had known for forty years had evaporated before her eyes. She seemed to accept these facts as they came, adjusting to each new level of decline. She never revealed any of her internal struggles. She grimly acquiesced to each new procedure without much question.

Sometimes I'd see her knitting bag with the pink scarf peeking out sitting alone on the chair next to Dr. Schwartz's bed. I'd find her in the solarium watching the boats on the East River. She didn't talk much with me, or anyone. "I just want him to get the tests so we can find out what's wrong," was about all she'd say, tucking a gray strand behind her ear. Her eyes drooped heavily, and they were closed a lot. Even when she appeared to be looking out at the boats.

I was deeply conflicted about Dr. Schwartz's medical management. If I were the attending, I would have sent him home on the very first day with arrangements for hospice care, an adequate supply of pain medications, and a DNR in his pocket. It seemed so simple.

But Dr. Schwartz was a patient of Dr. Gursky's—I was only the intern. It was Dr. Gursky's clinical judgment that determined the medical management. Dr. Gursky's approach was medically correct—I knew that—but it just didn't feel right. I longed to tell Mrs. Schwartz how I would handle the case, but it was an unwritten rule of UH: you never undermine the attending.

My one-month rotation at UH was thankfully drawing to a close. The diagnostic workup for Dr. Schwartz had been frustrated at every turn. Every attempt at a tissue diagnosis came up as "nondiagnostic," even though we all knew that the diagnosis was end-stage cancer of some type.

Dr. Schwartz was now only a shadow of his former self. Mrs. Schwartz was ever-more haggard appearing. The pink scarf hung lifeless from her knitting needles, having stopped growing long ago. I dragged my dilemma with me every day on rounds. To whom was my allegiance, the attending or the patient? Would I add to the confusion and worsen the situation for Mrs. Schwartz by tossing in my opinions and biases? Would I rankle the ire of the higher-ups and jeopardize my standing in the department? What would I want if that were my father in the hospital bed?

I was walking by Dr. Schwartz's room on one of my last days and noticed Mrs. Schwartz sitting silently, her shoulders hunched with fatigue, the knitting bag at her feet. Her right hand lay on the bed, just inches from her husband's mittened, restrained hand. Suddenly I forgot about the errand at hand and slipped impulsively inside the room. I sat close to Mrs. Schwartz and spoke in a low voice. I doubted if Dr. Schwartz could hear, much less comprehend, but I felt obliged to use discretion.

"Please don't tell Dr. Gursky that I've spoken to you, but I feel that you should know about other options that are available. Getting a tissue diagnosis is important but it is not paramount. Sometimes the overall clinical status of a patient provides a more accurate prognosis than the actual type of cancer."

It was almost too painful to look into the hooded, exhausted eyes of Mrs. Schwartz. "You don't have to do any of these treatments just because Dr. Gursky recommends them," I said. "You can take him home if you want, with home nursing or hospice care. You could take him home right now if you want, before the dinner trays come around." I paused, catching my breath. "He is dying of cancer no matter what we do."

There was a long silence. The air was heavy with antiseptic and I felt light-headed. The quiet made my stomach quiver, so I kept talking to fill the space. "Dr. Schwartz can't speak for himself now, but you know him better than we do. Our goal is to carry out what he would want, not what you or I or Dr. Gursky thinks should be done. If you could ask him now what he would want done, what do you think he would he say?"

Mrs. Schwartz sighed but didn't say anything. She picked up the dormant pink scarf and ran her fingers along the stitches. There was a fine set of white flowers along the edges that I hadn't noticed before. Mrs. Schwartz looked up at me briefly, then her gaze fell down to the gray linoleum. She continued in her silence.

"It's just that you should know—he doesn't have to do anymore of these tests."

"I think this is the right thing," Mrs. Schwartz said, raising her head slightly. "How could I give up if there's even the slimmest chance in the world? He would never give up without a fight. How could we abandon him?" Her fist tightened around the scarf. "How could *I* abandon him?"

She looked at me. Tears lined the rims of her eyes. "I'm sorry," I said softly, standing up and backing away. "Maybe you want to be alone."

I escaped from the room and found a chair in the solarium. Had I done the right thing? I felt guilty sneaking behind Dr. Gursky. But I also felt relieved—I had finally unburdened myself. An elderly woman eased herself into the chair next to me with the aid of a walker. A nurse's aide followed behind her, pushing her IV pole. She tucked the woman's robe around her waist and unfastened the top of a Jell-O container. She helped the woman manipulate her spoon into the container and guide the trembling orange glob into her mouth.

By the next week I was out of University Hospital and gratefully back at Bellevue. A few weeks later I decided to page Dr. Gursky and see how things had played out with Dr. Schwartz.

It turned out that they had been unable to make a tissue diagnosis with any of the multiple "external" methods they'd tried, so they took Dr. Schwartz to the operating room to attempt definitive diagnosis and treatment. His post-op course was complicated by cardiac arrhythmias and post-operative infections. He ended up in the intensive care unit where he suffered a cardiac arrest. He died after an unsuccessful resuscitation attempt. "By the way," Dr. Gursky added, "his family asked me to thank you. They really appreciated the care you provided."

I hung up the phone and put my head into my palms, rubbing my eyes heavily. I suddenly thought of Elba Rodriguez and her death in my first month of internship. I tried, I whispered. I tried to do it better. But Dr. Schwartz had died the miserable hospital death that I'd so dreaded. My intervention did nothing to alter the course of his demise, though maybe Mrs. Schwartz had made a more informed decision after our conversation.

Perhaps if Dr. Schwartz had presented to the hospital earlier in the course of his illness, the invasive procedures of the medical workup and the surgery could have offered him something. But he'd waited until he was literally on the verge of death.

I mulled over how a psychoanalyst could fall prey to such a primitive defense as denial. But maybe it wasn't so simple. Maybe he really knew what was happening as he got sicker and was aware what would happen once he deposited himself at the door of the hospital.

He may have forfeited the possibility of effective treatment by waiting so long, but perhaps he'd done that intentionally. Maybe he chose to give himself and his wife one last year of blissful "denial," one year free from the discomforts and indignities and exorbitant costs of medical care, one year devoid of constant worries, one year without the painful label of cancer. Perhaps he was far shrewder than I had imagined and had willfully cloaked his cognizance with a veil of denial. He may have seen to it that his wishes were indeed carried out, only letting the doctors in when he was good and ready to die. Perhaps he was helping me to tease out some of the finer points of medicine. Maybe Dr. Schwartz was being the true academic physician—steadfastly teaching and passing on "clinical pearls" to interns at every opportunity. Maybe he was trying to lend me a hand up that mountain. I only wish I'd taken the opportunity to ask him.

I had always relied on the dependability of institutional education. After all, I'd been in it for a good twenty years. From elementary school to medical school, clear-cut curricula were laid out, with defined endpoints and easily testable concepts. This system broke down in residency. While there was a formal noontime conference everyday, most learning was fragmented. Whether it was a tiny hint during attending rounds about how best to palpate the spleen, or a tip from a fellow resident about remembering the causes of metabolic acidosis, education now came in erratic bits like splattering raindrops. Sometimes the lessons were obvious, but other times, like with Dr. Schwartz, they were subtle and often took a long time to even notice, much less incorporate. And sometimes they didn't occur on rounds, or even in the hospital. Sometimes they turned up much closer to home, with friends from childhood, from a time way before I'd even thought about becoming a doctor.

CHAPTER SEVEN

The Burden of Knowledge

> If we'd been allowed to choose,
> we'd probably have gone on forever.
>
> Wisława Szymborska, "One Version of Events"

I HAD JUST STARTED medical school when Josh told me that he had IHSS. He offered to let me listen to his heart murmur with my brand-new stethoscope, but I declined. Josh was my buddy ever since we were eleven years old at summer camp in the Catskills. Our whole group of friends went to the same camp every year. Overnight hikes, lukewarm showers, tasteless food, mosquito-infested cabins— the summers were salvation from my bland high school. Josh always brought his guitar to camp and sang Pete Seeger and Phil Ochs songs. He played basketball and volleyball, but was a good sport about joining me in activities like folk dancing and singing. Between summers, Josh wrote me letters in all capital, block print. Always in red pen.

I visited Josh when he worked on a kibbutz in Israel after graduating college; he tracked me down whenever he was back in the States. Later, when he returned to New York, we remained close friends. We always ate at his favorite Indian restaurant on East Sixth Street, which he claimed was far superior to the other eleven Indian restaurants on the same block.

When medical school overwhelmed me, Josh would entertain me with stories of the eccentric characters in his graduate school library science program while chewing *chapatis* and *gulab jaman*. The owner always gave us free appetizers because he and Josh had once been waiters together.

Josh took me on a late-night tour of the ABC television newsroom where he worked as a researcher. He showed me where Ted Koppel broadcasted *Nightline* and I got to see the *Good Morning America* set.

I loved that Josh and I were about the same height. When we talked, we were always right at eye-level. Whenever he was ribbed about becoming a librarian—which happened a lot in our circle of friends—he would pull his glasses way down over his nose, stare out over the top with his mischievous brown eyes, and launch into an impassioned defense of the Dewey Decimal system.

Josh's father also had IHSS (idiopathic hypertrophic subaortic stenosis): a congenital thickening of the heart muscle. Josh's father had chest pain and shortness of breath and eventually required a heart transplant. Everyone knew that Josh's father had heart problems, but a lot of our friends weren't aware that Josh had the same condition. After all, Josh had played basketball and run track in high school. Because of the hereditary nature of the disease, his family was being followed by the National Institutes of Health. Periodically Josh would make the five-hour trip to Bethesda, Maryland, for ultrasounds, EKGs, and blood tests. The doctors were interested in how IHSS developed in members of a family. Josh confided to me, however, that he often skipped his appointments because the trip was too much of a hassle. Beyond that, Josh never talked much about the IHSS.

One Saturday night, late in the autumn of my internship year, I had tickets for a concert at Carnegie Hall with my best friend Rachel. We had invited Josh but he couldn't come because he was going to Mystic, Connecticut, for the weekend with his new girlfriend. Rachel and I went alone, gossiping about this new girlfriend and the prospects of something serious developing. Usually I didn't go out the night before being on call, but the a capella group Sweet Honey in the Rock was appearing for one night only at Carnegie Hall.

The next day, Sunday, I spent on call at Bellevue. I was exhausted from having stayed out late the night before, but I'd decided it was worth it. You had to live a little during internship, I told myself, otherwise you'd go crazy. When I arrived home at midnight after sixteen hours of work, my answering machine was blinking furiously with messages.

"Hi Danielle, this is Harold.... uh, call me when you get in," came the first message in a strangely expressionless voice.

"Danielle, this is Ari calling from Toronto. Can you ... umm ... call me?"

"It's Rosina in San Francisco. Please call me."

"Hi this is Laurie. It's six o'clock in Chicago now. Call when you get in."

"Danielle, it's Einat. Call me when you get in."

"It's Karen. I'm at my parents' house in Montreal. You can call late if you want to."

"Danielle, it's Willy. Ummm ... Call me."

And so the messages went. Each in a monotone voice, not leaving any message per se, but instructing me to call. The fifteenth message was from Rachel.

"Please call me when you get in. I'm staying on the Upper West Side. Call as late as you want."

My fingers were tingling when I dialed Rachel's number. Sit down Danielle, she said, when she answered the phone. Obediently I groped for a chair. She drew in a long breath and the phone static prickled my ears. Josh, she said, Josh had a cardiac arrest last night.

A cardiac arrest? Josh?

Josh and his girlfriend had been walking down the boardwalk in Mystic. When she turned to talk to him, he wasn't there. He had collapsed on the ground.

A cardiac arrest? Josh was only twenty-seven years old.

Emergency medical workers had arrived on the scene almost immediately. They tried to resuscitate him for more than thirty minutes.

My breath quivered, caught in my gullet.

They worked hard, they really did.

I could feel the layers of my skin curdle, disengaging from my body.

They kept going, they didn't want to give up.

The air thinned, depleting itself of oxygen.

They pronounced him dead.

The room trembled and its borders grew indistinct. Rachel's words pitched out of focus.

Stay right there, Danielle. I'm jumping into a taxi. I'll be there in ten minutes.

The room dissolved into silence.

Josh?

∽Only the forced routine of Bellevue kept me functioning as I slogged through the next day. Though I managed to follow my team down the endless hallways, my feet didn't register the ground. I had to remind myself which foot to put where.

I waded through my roster of patients. Who were they, anyway? What the hell were they doing here? Why didn't they all just go home?

Mrs. Chin. Lung cancer. Chemo starts tomorrow. Josh is dead?

Mr. Castaneda. Pneumonia. Needs a follow-up X-ray. Josh is dead?

Ms. Brewer. Endocarditis. Day five of nafcillin and gentamicin. Josh is dead?

My resident was willing to let me leave early for the funeral, but I still had to get my work done. My final task of the day was to place a central line—an extra-large IV in a central vein for long-term use. The young man who needed this central line was an end-stage AIDS patient. He was already on a ventilator and had been designated DNR by his mother. He had no semblance of consciousness left but was still plagued by infections. He needed antibiotics, but he was so swollen that the only place left to put in an IV was the broad femoral vein that coursed up the thigh into the groin. Four months of internship had made me a pro at central lines.

I prepped the site with iodine and local anesthetic. His thighs were swollen, but I was fairly sure that I could accurately detect the femoral pulse. The pulse of the femoral artery would tell me that the femoral vein was a mere fingerbreadth away. With two fingers secured on my landmark pulse, I slid the needle in. I focused on the plastic syringe, awaiting the triumphant flow of blood. Nothing came. I pulled out and tried again. No blood return. I rechecked the femoral pulse and adjusted my needle. Nothing. Josh, how could you leave me?

I ground my teeth and stabbed the needle again. Nothing. I mashed my fingers in the doughy flesh, hunting for the femoral pulse. When I was sure that I'd captured regular pulsations beneath my fingers, I jabbed the needle in. Nothing. Maybe those pulsations were just the pulse of my own fingers. My boundaries were beginning to tremble. Was this my pulse or his pulse? Josh, how could you die?

I bit my lip and sliced through the skin once again with my needle. Nothing. Just bloodless flesh of an inanimate body.

I wrenched the needle from the skin, re-aiming and firing again. Who are you, I screamed mutely at the legs in front of me. Why are you forcing me to stab this needle in? You are already comatose and dead—leave me alone. Why are you keeping me from Josh? I slammed the needle for the tenth and eleventh times, tears dripping into my sterile field.

My hair had slipped out from its band. Hot sticky tufts clumped on my neck, choking off the air. Brown iodine was splotched all over the front of my coat. Please, God, rescue me. Kill this man who is torturing me. Kill this man and let me go. Kill this man who is already dead and give me back my Joshua, who is supposed to be alive.

I stabbed and stabbed at the unyielding flesh, praying for the appearance of blood. A medical student walked by the door. "I need some help over here," I called out weakly. "Please get my resident in 16-West." When the student left the room, I gored the needle downward, not caring where it landed or what it destroyed. Blood suddenly flooded into my syringe. The heavy crimson of venous blood surged upward, heaving into the barrel of the syringe under the force of that still-clinging heart. The sight of blood, far from being nauseating as it might have been earlier in my life, was my very salvation. The dusky scarlet was a relief to my eyes, the palpable viscosity a balm to my fingers that were gripping the syringe. The muscles of my arms and my legs and my shoulders unclenched themselves as the blood poured forth. Oh God, thank you for this blood. This blood that is my deliverance.

Just before I dashed out, I turned back to look at the young man hooked up to the ventilator. He was about the same age as Josh. His body was drenched in sweat from his intractable fevers. His arms were black and blue from the endless IVs. His limbs were bloated from the fluids we were forcing into his veins. His eyes were caked closed with crumbly dried secretions, forced into oblivion, cast behind by the world that insisted on progressing without him. The room was silent except for the whir of the ventilator and the low-pitched grind of the IV machine. The sparkling view of the East River sat unused in the window, relentless shimmering of sun on water like actors without an audience. I froze at the door, one hand clutching the frame. His mother would hold his hand during her long lonely visits. Sometimes she read to him—novels, poems, magazines—whatever she had in her bag. "I'm sorry," I whispered. "I'm so sorry."

 More than two hundred people crowded into the synagogue, dazed and weeping. My friends from childhood—Rachel, Einat, Harold, Willy, Rosina; we sat in the wooden seats, looking back and forth at each other with the perplexed feeling that we had come to the wrong place. Funerals were supposed to be for old people, not for us. Not for Josh.

Friends and relatives got up and spoke about Josh. I recalled how I had helped him with his *PennySaver* paper route when we were twelve. He and I delivered papers all over his neighborhood, schlepping the heavy canvas sacks up and down the streets. It was June and we were hot and sweaty. Josh kept me entertained by doing imitations of his Hebrew School teacher who had a lisp and a facial twitch. When we finally finished we had accumulated several respectable dollars in tips. We debated what to do with our earnings—spend them now or deposit them in our bank accounts? At Josh's suggestion we trekked over to Friendly's and bought the largest ice cream sundae on the menu— three scoops with whipped cream, butterscotch, and walnuts. Two spoons, please. Was Josh thinking about his IHSS then?

The New Year's Eve that we'd spent in Israel. Josh was living in Haifa, studying at the Technion Institute. His apartment had no heat and it was freezing inside the ancient stone walls. We rigged up a strategic system with the single electric heater, two summer blankets, and his electric teapot so we could stay warm while playing an all-night back-gammon tournament. Was Josh thinking about his IHSS then?

I thought about when Josh had worked as a union organizer, traipsing through factories in the Midwest, talking with the workers. Was he thinking about his IHSS then? People shared stories—some touching, others hilarious. At times I laughed so hard that I choked on my tears.

Open caskets are generally not part of Jewish funerals, but there was a viewing before the service. Rachel and I could not bring ourselves to look. After the service, however, I was overcome with a pressing need to look. If I didn't look, if I didn't verify with my own eyes, I wouldn't believe that it was actually my Josh in that wooden box. This whole thing could very well be a hoax—Josh wasn't really dead. They were just burying an empty coffin. Later on, Josh would sneak up behind me with his irrepressible smile, peer out over his glasses, and say, "Fooled you!"

The funeral director lifted open the cover for us. Rachel and I held hands and held our breath. But there was Josh. It wasn't frightening at all; it was really him. Soft curly hair framed his sleeping face. His immaculate white shirt and pressed silk tie hid the autopsy scars. He had the beard that he had recently acquired with the thought of looking more grown-up. But he still looked like the little boy I'd delivered *PennySaver*s with. I reached in to finger the lapel of his gray wool suit. I remembered the wonderful surprise of running into Josh on Seventh Avenue and Seventeenth Street the day he'd bought that suit at Barney's autumn sale. It had only been a month ago.

After the service we went to Josh's parents' house to begin the week of *shiva*, the Jewish ritual of mourning. Most people gathered in clumps, physically grasping one another for support. Others wandered in erratic circles in the yard, circling near the wooden shed that Josh and his father had built, each spiraling in their own orbit. There was a sense of being shell-shocked, particularly for those who hadn't known about Josh's heart condition. I was one of only two doctors present. As an intern I was still adjusting to my role as a physician, still learning to respond when somebody said, "Dr. Ofri," still growing into my white coat. I was still feeling out my new muscles, unkinking and flexing them. I wasn't ready to represent and defend the world of medicine and the frustrating enigmas of the human body.

Struggling with the heavy words, I explained what IHSS was to each person who cornered me with their confusion and pain. "It's about the muscle that does the pumping," I would start, feeling the stiffness of clinical medicine elbowing into my grief. There was a vague relief in the terse roteness of the words—direct quotes from *Harrison's*—but I didn't want it clouding me, contaminating this space, weighing in on my sadness. I didn't want the responsibility and burden of medicine. I wanted to wander in the yard and cry. I wanted to slump against the wooden shed in the backyard and collapse my limbs against it. I wanted to relinquish the aching effort it took just to stand upright to the wordless comfort of the pine planks. But over and over I described the clinical manifestations of IHSS. I held back my tears and recited words about the left ventricle and the aortic valve and the risk of ar-rhythmias. I wanted to go outside and touch that shed, touch the wood that Josh's hands had held, that his hands had nailed and sanded and sawed. I wanted to inhale its musty solace. But instead I patiently an-swered questions about cardiac arrest and resuscitation. I tried to be as delicate as possible. I even found myself saying that a patient in a cardiac arrest dies without feeling much pain. I was trying not to worsen anyone's grief, but I knew that I wasn't telling the truth.

*∽*I hate codes.

The dramatic, sanitized versions of cardiac arrests, or "codes," on television bear little resemblance to reality. A real-life code is an anar-chy of people yelling, IVs messily inserted, iodine splattering, rubber gloves and blood-soaked gauze flying about, reams of EKG paper spilling endlessly onto the floor, the smell of singed flesh after 360-kilojoule shocks. It is brutally physical. If you don't break some ribs then you haven't done effective CPR—so the intern's saying goes. The thought of my beloved Josh dying in this manner broke my heart. I couldn't bear to tell any of my fellow mourners the truth about codes.

Codes are almost always futile because they usually occur in people who are gravely ill, people like Dr. Schwartz who are sick enough that their hearts cease beating. In the event someone is "brought back," their brains have usually been without oxygen for so long that there is significant brain damage. Their lives are back, but their personalities and consciousness are gone. And usually the illness that made them sick enough to have a cardiac arrest is still there, just waiting to kill them a few days or weeks later.

Ever so rarely, when there is a dramatic save of a person with a treatable illness, a reasonably healthy life can be restored. I suppose that is what keeps us going through this morbid ritual of CPR. Nonetheless, I have signed a living will saying that I do not ever want to be resuscitated in this manner if I have a terminal illness. Just crank up my morphine.

The most surreal aspect for me when I run a code is determining the time of death. The time of death is not recorded as the time when the patient was found to be unresponsive, without a pulse, blood pressure, or respirations (i.e., dead). No, the patient is only dead when I decide that the code is over. The official time that appears on the death certificate is the time on my watch when I utter that understated but universally accepted euphemism, "Thank you very much, everybody, for your help." With those bland words the furious activity comes to a screeching halt. The monitors are turned off, the ventilator is silenced, the IVs are clamped, and everybody shrinks away from this altar of death, piled high with the offerings of medical science. Only the nurse's aides remain to remove the detritus of our "resuscitation," carefully cleaning the body to erase the indignities of a medically attended death.

I had been assured in Josh's case that the medics had gotten there immediately, that no time had been lost in starting the code. But deep inside I had my doubts. He could just as easily have been with me at the concert that night instead of out on the boardwalk. What if he'd had his cardiac arrest sitting next to me, a physician and friend who loved him dearly? Could I have done a faster, better job? Could I have resuscitated him right there on the red velvet seats of Carnegie Hall? Could that few-seconds advantage I would have had over even the fastest ambulance have made a difference? Or was I overinflating my abilities, indeed the abilities of the medical profession.

I've laid awake many nights dissecting this scenario in agonizing detail. The grand ceiling of Carnegie Hall, under which, only a few months ago, I had marched in my black robe with the regal purple velvet trim. The silken hood draped around my neck—green lining for the doctorate of medicine, gold stripe for the doctorate of philosophy in science. The gilded stage upon which I'd received my diploma. The hall from which we had recited the oath of Hippocrates and the code of Maimonides. "... For the mind of man is puny, and the art of healing vast ..."

That same hall could have held Josh on that night, had he chosen to attend the concert with me instead of going to Mystic. My fingers burned with the feeling of his skin growing cold against mine. My mouth against his, forcing desperate air in. My hands on his chest, pumping, pounding, railing at his heart to beat.

Would I have been able to conduct a code in the narrow space between the rows of red velvet seats? Would I have remembered the resuscitation protocols? Or would I have been paralyzed with fear and simply unable to act?

And the music. Would the music have kept playing?

℘Several months later I was working overnight in the cardiac care unit. Mr. Cronley was a man in his early thirties with IHSS. He had been plagued by dizziness and fainting spells as well as the memories of three young family members who had died of sudden cardiac arrest. In the morning he was to undergo a procedure to eradicate the irregular heart rhythm presumably responsible for his symptoms as well as his family members' deaths.

It was nearly three A.M. and he was sitting bolt upright in his chair, tangled in a morass of wires linking him to multiple monitors. He was paralyzed by the fear of sudden cardiac death, too afraid to move or even go to sleep. I wanted to comfort him, to allay his terrors, but I was burdened by my medical knowledge and my own unhealed grief. How could I reassure Mr. Cronley that the medical profession would make him better? I didn't have the strength to be the empathic physician. I felt too young and too small to carry this burden. If this was what it meant to be a doctor—to allow my patient to collapse the weight of his fears against me, while juggling my own pains that lunged relentlessly at my ballast—I didn't think I was strong enough. I wasn't sure if I would ever be strong enough. I was burdened with memories that still clawed at my own heart, so I couldn't reassure my patient about his. I could only think about Josh. Josh delivering papers with me and sharing an ice cream sundae. Josh singing old union songs on his guitar at camp. Josh lying between the red velvet seats at Carnegie Hall.

When my patient's fear-laden eyes caught mine, I could only look down. I could only feel my legs tremble and threaten to give out beneath me. I could only mumble some platitudes that I hoped sounded reasonable and escape as soon as possible, feeling wretched.

℘Our medical training has always reinforced the belief that knowledge is power. One could always be stronger with more facts at hand. Knowledge provides the girders and buttresses of the medical edifice. Now I'm not so sure. Years have passed since Josh's death. My friends and I still miss him painfully. I think about the hikes we took together in the Catskill Mountains during our summers, how Josh always noticed the details of rock formations on the trail, how he always managed to have extra water in his canteen, how he loved to light a "one-match" campfire with just the right ratio of birchbark, twigs, and sticks balanced in a pyramid. I cry every time I've reread the words of this chapter, every time I've corrected a spelling error or added a semicolon or adjusted a margin. From the first scribbled words on the back of a used manila envelope at four o'clock in the morning after yet another panicked dream about Josh, to the eleventh and fifteenth rewrites, to the final proof of the galleys just before publication, the tears always flow. It never seems to get easier. And beyond the aching emptiness created by his absence, I feel the extra agony of knowing the sound of cracking ribs during resuscitation, the feel of slammed-in breathing tubes, the sight of splattering blood from IVs. I am tormented by the nightmare of Josh sitting beside me at Carnegie Hall, and what I could, or could not, have done.

And then I am haunted by the perhaps even more horrendous possibilities had he been "successfully" resuscitated. Might I now, instead of remembering Josh on his *yartzheit*—the anniversary of his death—be visiting his vegetative body in a nursing home? I shudder to think of him condemned to years of respirators and tube feedings—bedsores and infections gradually gnawing away at his beautiful young body. The burden of knowledge extends even further back to that day, years ago, when a lump grew in my throat as Josh told me of his IHSS and casually offered to let me listen to his heart murmur. I couldn't bear to listen. I couldn't bear to verify the impending burden.

℘Next to my bed stands a picture of Josh and me, aged fourteen, at summer camp. We have our arms casually slung around each other's shoulders and the camera caught the golden slanting sunlight of a late August afternoon. In the photo we are both gazing off into the distance, serious expressions on our faces. I remember that we were posing, pretending to look sophisticated and grown-up. I'm not sure what was on my mind at that time, but it certainly wasn't medicine or IHSS. I'm sure we were thinking about the pleasures of summer, with the languid reassurance of long August days. I'm sure we were basking in the warmth of endless possibilites, unburdened by knowledge yet to come.

THE INTERN WAS NEARLY IN TEARS. "I can't go back in that guy's room," Sarita sniffled. "I've been trying to get an IV in for almost an hour, and he won't stop yelling at me. But he doesn't have any veins."

I had been an intern, or first-year resident, only last month, but now that July 1st had rolled around again, I was a second-year resident. As a second-year resident, I had to supervise and teach my own team of interns. When I was an intern I'd had to do all the horrible scut work for my patients, but I always had the relief of my resident, who made all the important decisions. No matter how awful things became, there was always my resident to turn to who seemed to know all the answers. Once the clock had struck 12:01 A.M. on July 1st, I had to come up with those answers myself.

I consulted my freshly printed index cards. Harold Goode—homeless, shooter with a fever, admitted last night, empiric antibiotics for possible endocarditis. I had picked up the 16-West service this morning and didn't know the patients yet, but I had to learn them quickly. Now I was the resident.

Sarita was biting her lip to keep from crying outright. Just last month she'd been a medical student and now she was an intern. This could be one of her very first IVs on her own. I remembered how difficult IVs were when I'd started residency as a night-float intern. I remembered that miserable sinking feeling when the needle pierced the skin and was met, yet again, with nothingness. The hatred toward the patient whose veins were too thin or too knobby or too scarred or too invisible. That would be when I'd page my resident, face flushed, neck clammy, and stammer out my failure, trying hard to sound casual. My resident would tell me not to worry about it, then walk into the room with unflappable calm and slip in an 18-gauge IV without spilling a drop of blood.

I hadn't been given any crash course on how to be a resident in charge. But it was the usual July 1st syndrome in which everyone was punted forward a notch. Like newborn piglets we wobbled forward into our new roles because there was no way to turn back the momentum. An intern was now standing before me in tears, entirely relying on me to save the day.

Me?

Sarita swallowed hard to keep her composure. Stipples of crimson crept through her dark olive skin as she fiddled fretfully with the reflex hammer that was hanging out of her second buttonhole. Born and raised in Madras in southern India, she'd moved to the United States for medical school. Though she was fully schooled in the "American way," as she liked to say, she still retained a faint British accent and some formal Indian mannerisms. As if she suddenly noticed her hands misbehaving, Sarita quickly tucked the hammer back in its place and straightened out her white coat, which was still crisp and pressed from the laundry service. Sarita's freshly minted ID card dangled from her right lapel and the smooth lamination glinted under the fluorescent lights. I glanced down at mine and suddenly noticed fingerprint smudges over my picture and particles of dirt that had gummed up the corners of the plastic holder. The edges had roughened, revealing the layers of plastic that had been pressed together to form the card. I was amazed that my ID card, which had so recently been momentously new with those brisk weighty letters "MD" after my name, had now acquired a worn look. A look of experience. A whole year had gone by and my ID card now looked experienced.

Did I look experienced?

Sarita was standing before me, inexplicably calming down as the burden of Mr. Goode shifted from her to me. Didn't she know that I'd been a measly intern just last week?

When in doubt, pretend. There didn't appear to be any other option.

I rolled the kinks out of my shoulders, pulled my back high, and started walking down the hall. Sarita trailed behind me. I sucked in my cheeks and strode into Mr. Goode's room with what I hoped was a look of authority.

"What seems to be the problem here?"

Mr. Goode was a man in his early thirties with a deep scowl etched into his face. He was about six feet tall with blunt, square shoulders. The sleeves of the blue patient gown strained from the bulk of his arm muscles. He looked surprisingly robust for an IV drug user living on the streets. "That little girl-doctor over there been stickin' me with needles," he said, pointing at Sarita. "She don't know what the fuck she doin'. Get me a real doctor." Sarita pulled her lips inward and dropped her gaze to the floor.

"Listen, Mr. Goode," I said with deliberate patience. "Dr. Singh is your doctor. If she has to put an IV in, you have to let her do it. You have a fever from shooting up drugs. This could be just a "hot shot" from dirt in the needle, but it could also be something much more serious. If your heart valves are infected, you're going to need six weeks of intravenous antibiotics." I added more heft to my voice. "And if you don't get the full treatment for endocarditis, you could get very sick. You might end up having open-heart surgery to replace the valves." I paused deliberately, waiting for a reaction to my well-crafted scare-tactics. He didn't budge. "You need an IV."

"Well, I want someone who knows what the hell they doin'." I could see Sarita's head dropping lower, until her chin was almost on her collar.

I swallowed hard and focused my eyes on the vitals chart at the foot of the bed to get away from his stare. "I'm in charge here. I'll put in the IV."

He smirked. "You in charge? What are you, an intern or somethin'? I don't want no first-year intern poking around my body with needles."

Did he know that July 1st had been the switch date? Or would he have said that to anybody? The other patients on my service seemed to accept me as the team leader without much question. I took in a deep breath and exhaled it slowly, trying to give myself time to regroup. When in doubt, I told myself, pretend. This time I looked right at him. I knew that Sarita was behind me and I didn't want to back down. "I'm the resident in charge," I said sharply. "I'll put in the IV."

Without waiting for a reply, I reached over and grasped his arm firmly, one hand around his wrist, the other at his elbow—a grasp, I hoped, that conveyed conviction. I surveyed the rich brown of his skin, hoping to see that faint greenish tinge that hints of freely flowing blood beneath the surface. I palpated his extremities for the subtle change in surface tension, the ever-so-slight variation in pliancy that indicates a vein, even if not visible to the eye. But no, his skin was unyielding. What veins were discernible were irrevocably scarred from previous use.

I went through the routine of turning his arm this way and that, looking for the "intern's vein" on the side of the wrist and the "secret vein" on the back of the forearm. I thwacked his arm with the back of my hand and I scoured his skin with alcohol swabs, but his vessels were inscrutable. Sarita had lifted her head slightly and was watching me in silence.

Last week I would have continued with intern doggedness. I would have kept poking at the increasingly futile veins: the evanescent ones on the inner surface of the wrist, the fickle ones on the fingers, the dubious ones on the web of the thumb, the precarious ones on the calves, the capricious ones on the foot. I would have kept going because my resident had instructed me to put in an IV and as an intern I was programmed to carry out my tasks.

But now there was no one telling me what to do. *I* was making the decision about the IV. Instead of endless stabbing with the needle I could actually step back and ask, "Does Mr. Goode truly need an IV; could this medication be given orally? Does he, in fact, even need this antibiotic at all?" As a resident, I had the prerogative to replace an IV torture session with dispassionate clinical decision-making skills. I could feel a tiny smile creeping up in my cheeks. Maybe this resident stuff wouldn't be so hard after all. Maybe you just started acting like you knew the answers and then you'd discover you actually knew them!

I reviewed the data in my head. Mr. Goode had been admitted last night with a fever and was being given antibiotics for possible endocarditis. Unlike Herbert Ziff, he didn't have already-damaged valves that would put him at extremely high risk for infection. Mr. Goode's EKG was normal and his vital signs were stable. He had no other textbook signs of endocarditis: heart murmur, Janeway lesions, Osler nodes, or Roth spots. His blood cultures were safely cooking in the microbiology lab. It would be perfectly appropriate, I reasoned, to withhold antibiotics and institute "watchful waiting" until the results of his blood cultures became available. Yeah, I thought, this is it. I could use my clinical experience to pursue reasoned, thoughtful judgment instead of wrestling with task-oriented intern tenacity. Being a resident wasn't so bad after all. I concentrated on the impression I would make on Sarita. Maybe she would look at me the way I'd viewed Li-Chan, or Miguel. They always seemed to have rich clinical facts at their disposal to teach me. Now I would have a chance to pass it on. I nodded to myself with satisfaction.

"Mr. Goode, I think we'll hold off on antibiotics for the moment—until the cultures come back. Then we'll decide whether you need antibiotics. And if the cultures are positive, we'll be able to choose the precise antibiotic because we'll know exactly which organism we're treating." Yes—reasoned, thoughtful judgment. I hoped Sarita was catching everything. I remembered how hard it was as an intern to take in everything at once.

Mr. Goode screwed up his face at me. "What the fuck you talkin' about, girl? When I stayed at Beth Israel they gave me antibiotics round the clock. What kind of shit doctors do they stick in Bellevue?"

My legs suddenly felt a little shaky. But I was the resident in charge, damn it, and I was going to stick to my clinical decision. "Well, right now we can't be sure that you actually have endocarditis," I said, "but we've done all the appropriate blood cultures." Reasoned thoughtful judgment.

"Get me some real doctors. You don't know shit."

"Mr. Goode, we are going to pursue clinical observation until we have microbiological confirmation." I hoped Sarita couldn't hear the ragged cadence in my voice.

"What kinda shit you talkin' about?" Mr. Goode sputtered, pushing himself forward on the bed so that his glare was even more focused at me. "You guys don't know what the fuck you doing. I gotta get me back to Beth Israel."

I edged one hand into a pocket, searching for familiar objects—my stethoscope, my reflex hammer, my penlight. Was it so obvious that I was sliding by the seat of my pants?

"Clinical observation is a perfectly acceptable way to treat suspected endocarditis." I begged my vocal cords to emit stronger, more commanding tones, but they felt tattered and hoarse. "After all, we don't even know for sure that you actually have it. There can be bad side effects, you know, to taking antibiotics if you don't actually need them."

Mr. Goode snorted and looked toward the window. I shifted my weight a few times, reshuffling the reflex hammer and the penlight. How was Sarita taking all of this? Did I look like an utter idiot? Mr. Goode continued to stare at the smokestacks from the factories in Queens across the river. The silence was leaden and clammy. I edged my way to the door hoping he wouldn't turn back to me. He didn't.

∽That night was Liver Rounds—one of the designated nights for residents to go out to a local bar and inflict damage upon their livers. I gazed at the motley housestaff swigging beers and laughing over chips and war stories. On the one hand, they were remarkably homogeneous—all high-achievers in their college and medical school classes, mostly middle class, white. The scheduling of residency, however, made people who would normally not ever socialize spend more time together than they would with even their spouses. This led to some interesting pairings. There was Mary, the born-again Christian who toted her pet iguana to every conceivable function, who worked with Jeremy, the orthodox Jew who kept kosher salami in his locker so he wouldn't have to eat in the cafeteria. There was Arun, the quiet Cambodian who had come to the United States on an illegal boat at age six, working with Simon, the brash Hungarian capitalist who frantically checked his stock quotes between admissions. Though there were many residents hailing from privileged homes with BMWs to spare, I learned there were probably equal numbers who had worked their way up, from working-class families in Brooklyn, or repressive systems in Shanghai.

My nervousness from the day was still rattling around in my chest. I eyed the residents who packed the bar, wondering who I could turn to—for what I wasn't even quite sure—but they all seemed so jolly and self-assured, hands comfortably curled around beer bottles, bodies loose and insouciant. Weren't they also nettled by the remaining shards of their day in the hospital, or could they shake it off so easily, like water in your hair when you popped out from a swimming pool for air?

The beer was disgusting, cheap brew for a large crowd. I nibbled on some broken pretzels that remained at the bottom of a well-scoured bowl—residents never passed up an opportunity for free food, no matter how meager. The pretzels were chalky and tasteless and the salt burned my chapped lips. I continued chewing on them for lack of anything better to do while the noise and festivities swirled around me. Everybody else seemed to be enjoying the weak beer and the stale pretzels. What was I missing?

We had barely begun rounds the next morning when the microbiology lab called. "Four out of four bottles, gram positive cocci!" a Russian accent barked over the phone. All of Mr. Goode's blood cultures had grown bacteria. So much for watchful waiting.

When Sarita and I arrived at Mr. Goode's bedside I explained the turn of events and the necessity for an IV. Mr. Goode cocked his head and narrowed his eyes at me. "So, you telling me that you bastards screwed up? I should've gone to Beth Israel. You assholes made me miss last night's antibiotics when I really needed them. I know how this shit works. I been around."

I explained my theory of watchful waiting, how I hadn't wanted to give him unnecessary medications, but now they were necessary, and now we needed to get an IV in, but lucky for him, and lucky for us, it was morning and the IV team was here so we—he—could benefit from the superior skills of the IV nurses. I wanted desperately to keep my clinical composure in front of Sarita, but my words stumbled over each over as my medical logic crumbled under Mr. Goode's fierce stare.

Later that afternoon when Sarita and I were rounding, I was both shamed and relieved to see that the IV team had managed to get a scrawny IV in his arm. "Look at this one, baby." Mr. Goode flaunted it at us. "You doctors don't know shit about IVs. I been around. I been to Beth Israel. I know what's up and I'll be stickin' with the IV team."

Sarita looked away hurriedly, pulling her index cards from her pocket and shuffling them haphazardly. I think she was trying to spare me the embarrassment. How I wished I could have sunk a 14-gauge IV into his deep brachial vein just at that moment. A really big, painful IV the size of a ballpoint pen—one stick, ram it in, no blood spilled. One solid IV barreling through all those scars and skin ulcers down to the damn obstreperous veins that I knew were lurking underneath his opaque, dark skin.

Stay calm, I told myself. Don't get into a power struggle with him in front of the intern. "I'm glad they got the IV in," I said, striving for the vaguely saccharine professional demeanor I'd heard attendings use. "Now you'll be able to get the medicine that you need." I spun around and strode out the door. Sarita grabbed her cards and scurried to catch up.

By nightfall the IV was out. Mr. Goode refused to let the night-float intern place one. The IV team came again the next morning. This time they managed to thread a pediatric IV into the edge of one of his jagged skin ulcers. It was out within a few hours.

"Mr. Goode," I said, "you need to have an IV in place all the time. You need four doses of nafcillin and three doses of gentamicin every day."

Mr. Goode was sitting up in bed. There was a pack of Marlboros, a bag of potato chips, and an open can of Dr. Brown's Cream Soda in his lap. "I be taking the IV, but I ain't letting no doctor put it in. I'll wait for the IV team." He took a swig of soda.

"The IV team is only here in the mornings. If the IV falls out during the afternoon, you have to let Dr. Singh replace it. If it falls out at night, the night-float intern will put it in."

"Listen, girl," he said, pointing his finger at me, "I ain't taking no shit from nobody. I don't want no Singh-shing-ding touching me. Ain't nobody putting no IV in me except the IV team. You got that?"

I took a half step back and found myself up against the window. Mr. Goode's finger was still piercing the air. Sarita looked nervously at me. I waited a moment until I felt more collected. "Mr. Goode," I said, controlling my voice as much as I could, "I know this is all very painful. I know that you feel sick now, but it is so important for you to get these antibiotics. Otherwise your heart valves could be destroyed."

"What do you know?" he sneered. "You don't know nothin'."

I felt a sting in my eyes. "For your information, Mr. Goode, I have treated a lot of patients with endocarditis, and I've seen how sick they can get." Mr. Goode dug his hand into the bag of potato chips and crammed a fistful into his mouth. Crumbs gathered on the edges of his lips and spilled onto his blue hospital gown. "I think we should consider putting in a central line," I continued. "That's a long IV catheter that goes into one of the body's larger veins in the neck or the thigh. It lasts for two weeks and can also be used to draw blood."

"I know what a goddamn central line is. You think I'm stupid?" Mr. Goode crumpled the bag of chips closed and pulled out a cigarette from the pack of Marlboros. "I been around. You ain't giving me no central line."

"Mr. Goode, there's no smoking in the hospital."

"I ain't taking none of your central lines. I be sticking with the IV team. They know what they doing." He struck a match and lit his cigarette. Sarita edged for the door.

"Mr. Goode, there are oxygen lines in these rooms. They could explode."

"Well hunky dory," he said taking a long drag and blowing the smoke in my direction.

I wet my parched lips with my tongue. "Mr. Goode," I said, pacing my words as evenly as I could, "you need to put out that cigarette."

"Go fuck yourself, bitch."

Sarita was already at the door, leaning tightly against the frame. I wanted to spit at him. I wanted to claw that cigarette from those obnoxious hands and stamp it out on the ground. I wanted to scream at him and tell him what a bastard he was. But under his glare I felt impotent. My knowledge and experience didn't seem to count for anything. I stomped out of the room and down the hall with Sarita scurrying behind me. I barked at one of the nurses, "Call security, damn it." That cigarette was going to get put out.

That night I had trouble sleeping. Mr. Goode's face popped into my dreams, leering at me with a twisted, ugly expression. His eyes practically spit acid at me as he'd say, "You don't know nothin', girl." And I began to hate him. I hated him for embarrassing me in front of Sarita. I hated him for knowing that "watchful waiting" had been a cop-out on my part. I hated him for understanding the hospital hierarchy and knowing that I'd been an intern only last week. I hated him for knowing just how terrified I was at the responsibility of being a doctor.

One day on rounds Mr. Goode was gone. Sarita smiled the first smile I'd seen all month. The entire floor breathed a collective sigh of relief. Happily at Beth Israel, I thought.

Unfortunately, Mr. Goode returned to Bellevue the very next day. And due to the "bounce-back" rule, he bounced right back to my team. On the day of his reappearance, Mr. Goode was even more irritable. He made offensive sexual remarks to the nurses and intimidated the housekeeper, who was too afraid to put sheets on his bed.

"What trash-hole you get that dress from," was how he greeted me when I entered his room that day.

Mr. Goode had arrived back on the ward sporting a microscopic IV next to his pinkie finger, obviously placed by some determined ER intern. It didn't make it through the first dose of gentamicin.

I presented the central line option once again to Mr. Goode, reminding him of the potential damage to his heart valves if his infection wasn't adequately treated. He wanted to continue with the IVs placed by the IV team. "At least they can get one in," he said. I told him that daily IVs placed on the edges of his skin ulcers lasting only three hours were not a realistic option for six weeks. He still refused the central line.

"Well," I said, "the only other choice is intramuscular injections of the antibiotics."

"In the arm, right?" he asked. I shook my head smugly, hoping Sarita would catch the meaning.

The nurse arrived with the first dose: four syringes of nafcillin. Mr. Goode glowered at her while she opened the alcohol wipes. I was surprised when he acquiesced to lowering the left side of his pants to allow her to clean the skin. She grasped a handful of his muscle and poised the first needle. "Okay, a little pinch now. One, two ..."

She hadn't gotten past two when Mr. Goode shrieked. The nurse persevered and plunged the needle all the way in.

"How many of those things you planning on stabbing me with?" he said, yanking his pants up.

"It's four syringes for a full dose. Every four hours to keep on schedule."

"What the fuck you all talking about?" He whirled around, hand still clutching his pajama bottoms. The nurse jumped back defensively. "Take your goddamn needles and your goddamn doctors out with you. Get the fuckin' IV team over here."

∽Whenever the IV team managed to get a tiny IV in Mr. Goode's arm, he was sure to point it out to us. "You doctors ain't worth shit," he said, cradling his IV like a medal of courage.

I examined the IV, angry that the IV team was almost making it harder for us by succeeding in placing an IV each day. I wanted to tell them to stop, but of course I couldn't. And the IVs never lasted anyway. This one was already leaking. "Mr. Goode, this IV is not sufficient for your antibiotics. Look at the leak."

"Well if you doctors are so smart, why don't you fix it?"

"Sarita," I said, "do you have some surgical tape?"

Sarita fished a roll out of her pocket and tore off three thin strips. I had expected her to hand the tape to me so I could retape the IV, but she started applying the strips herself, looping the sticky tape around the head of the IV.

Mr. Goode leaned in close as she taped the second and third layers on. His voice lowered. "In some countries they sell dark girls like you to the highest bidder." I shook my head, not sure if I'd heard correctly. Sarita's fingers were still affixed to the tape; she couldn't dislodge her hands immediately, but I could see them tremble. "But I don't know if they'd take you," Mr. Goode added.

At that Sarita sprang back—the tape and the IV came along with her and a trail of blood dribbled down Mr. Goode's arm from the IV site. I grabbed Sarita by the arm and pulled her out of the room with me.

"Goddammit," I said out loud to the air while Sarita sank back against the wall blinking back tears. "I hate that man, I hate him."

When Mr. Goode eloped the next day, I treated my entire team to breakfast at the coffee shop. And brought back extra glazed donuts for the nurses.

∽The next Thursday Mr. Goode was re-admitted to my service. I begged the medical consult to give him to another team but apparently there were at least three "frequent fliers" in the ER, and each team had to get one—the Bellevue rule.

I steeled myself before I went to see him, awaiting the barrage that would greet me as soon as he recognized me. But Mr. Goode didn't act surprised at all to see me. It was as though we hadn't missed a beat and this was simply the next day. "I'm tired of all you people's shit. Next time I be going to Beth Israel Hospital. They got real doctors at Beth Israel." I almost had to smile at his efficiency, dispensing with the unnecessary greetings and medical history.

Taking him up on his cue, I cut right to the heart of the matter. "You have endocarditis, Mr. Goode. You need a central line."

"No way. I don't want your damn central line," he said, methodically tearing to bits a 4x4 gauze pad. "You'd probably pop my lungs on the way in."

So far I hadn't yet deflated anyone's lungs from putting in a central line, but I was terrified that I might. How did Mr. Goode always know just what my fears were? "Mr. Goode," I said, "you can die from this infection. It can kill you if it's not treated. Getting only a few doses of medicine per day is not enough to treat the infection."

He let the scraps of gauze flutter onto his bedsheets. "I don't want your fucking central line. I know the IV team here; they can get me an IV."

I folded my hands across my chest, determined to stand my ground, knowing that I was right. "Intermittent antibiotic dosing will actually make things worse. It might kill some bacteria, but it will leave behind those strains that are resistant to the antibiotics. The mortality rate for antibiotic-resistant endocarditis is extremely high."

Mr. Goode looked down at his hands and flicked some dirt off his fingernails. "All right, girl," he said slowly. Then he looked up and thrust one wagging finger in my face. "But I don't want to feel no pain. You better give me something for the pain. I don't like them needles."

Didn't like needles? How'd he manage his career as an IV drug addict?

I promised him adequate local anesthesia but warned him that he still might feel some discomfort. I assured him that it would be very transient and urged him to focus on the two weeks of benefits rather than the few unpleasant moments.

I laid out the materials for the central line, trying hard to conceal the syringe with the metallic four-inch needle from Mr. Goode's view while I cleaned and sterilized his skin. I kept the needle at a low angle as I maneuvered it toward the site of entry, hoping he wouldn't notice its size, but Mr. Goode sat up with a start. He took a hard and nasty look at the needle in my hand and his eyes began to bug out. He lurched off the bed and pulled his body up to its fullest height. I stepped back instinctively.

"I'll give you one stick, girl," Mr. Goode hissed. His hot breath shot undiminished toward my face. The needle glinted in my hand, its reflection incongruously sparkly and festive.

I surveyed the track marks on his arms and the ragged craters of his skin ulcers. I considered the various viruses that were probably circulating in his bloodstream. I looked back at the needle.

"I don't want to be feeling nothing," Mr. Goode said, his upper lip curling inward as he stared straight at me. Shadows crawled down the sides of his cheekbones.

I reflected on my offer to Mr. Goode of short-term discomfort in exchange for long-term gain. I considered the authority my words carried by virtue of being a physician—a resident in charge. I looked back at the needle.

"I'll give you one stick," Mr. Goode repeated, "and if I feel anything, anything, I'll be goin' off on you!" The extra puff of air he spewed with his final words bathed me in a bitter combination of tobacco smoke and unbrushed teeth. I glanced at the enormous needle in my hand. I didn't even know what "goin' off" on somebody meant, but I didn't want to find out.

Something tightened and shuddered uncontrollably inside me.

I bit down on my lip and dumped the needle in the sharps disposal. I gathered the rest of the central line kit and swept it into the garbage pail. My hand trembled as I wrote a prescription for oral antibiotics. "Here are your pills, Mr. Goode," I said in a quivering but audible voice. "You can leave the hospital in the morning." I corralled every muscle fiber I possessed to walk calmly out the door. As soon as I was out of view from Mr. Goode, I staggered into the nurses' station. I collapsed into a chair in the corner and pretended to read the temperature charts so that no one would notice the shaking.

I had never thrown anyone out of the hospital. I'd never given up on a patient before. I'd never hated a patient before. I hadn't realized that being in charge might entail denying my patients medical care. Sending a man who had an infection of his heart valves out of the hospital with a couple of pills was a far cry from the "standard of care." A deep-seated infection like endocarditis would never respond to the relatively weak oral antibiotics—but what could I do?

❧A year and a half later, I was on call one night as the medical consult, the person in charge of admitting patients to the medical service.

I was paged to the recovery room at two A.M. to see a post-op patient in renal failure who was not recovering from anesthesia. Could I please evaluate this patient and transfer him from the surgical service to the medical intensive care unit? I trudged through the deserted eleventh floor with my fifth cup of coffee and blearily pushed through the automatic double doors.

The recovery room was lined with post-op patients in various states of consciousness, but I spotted him immediately. I blinked a few times to make sure I was seeing clearly, but there was Mr. Goode. A small shudder rippled involuntarily in my stomach at the very sight of him. Just seeing him there, even half-asleep, brought back memories of that intimidating sneer, of the way he could make me feel so inconsequential, of him swaggering at me over the central line needle.

He had the same imposing body, but this time it was riddled with medical paraphernalia: a breathing tube emerged from his mouth, two chest tubes emanated from his rib cage, a bright yellow Swan-Ganz catheter entered his neck and snaked all the way through his heart chambers to his lungs, a Foley catheter collected his urine, a dialysis catheter exited the femoral artery in the groin, a nasogastric tube traveled from his nose into his stomach. The cloth restraints on his arms were a testament to the battle he managed to wage with the nurses even in his semiconscious state.

I leafed through his hefty chart and beheld a chronicle of medical care stymied by anger. He had been on the medical service for the past several weeks with his umpteenth bout of endocarditis. Numerous notes reported "patient refusing IVs," "patient uncooperative with staff," "patient verbally threatening to nurses," "patient throwing food tray at roommate," "patient harassing medical students," "patient left hospital during the night," "patient returned, cocaine noted in urine tox."

The notes evinced progressive exasperation until there was an abrupt change of tone: "patient with persistent fever," "patient noted to have dropping blood pressure," "patient complaining of shortness of breath," "patient with increasing weakness." Fluid gathered around his heart like it had done with Zalman Wiszhinsky, compressing its chambers. In Mr. Goode's case, however, rampant infection caused the fluid to solidify. The fluid could not be removed with a simple needle drainage; surgery was the only option.

To the end, Mr. Goode remained his obnoxious self. He consented to and then refused surgery several times. The cardiac surgeons and anesthesiologists were increasingly irritated as the operation was repeatedly scheduled and then postponed. As well, Mr. Goode's window of opportunity for intervention was rapidly closing as the fluid evolved into a fibrous mass.

After several rounds, the surgeons took his next consent at face value and declined to acknowledge his subsequent protestations. Mr. Goode insisted on "feeling absolutely nothing" not just during the surgery, but also during the elevator ride down to the operating room. Even with sedation to keep him woozy, Mr. Goode could not stop complaining. Under heavy doses of sedative he managed to pull out his IV and call the orderly a "nigger prick." "I don't want to be feelin' no pain," he said. "I be takin' off if this stuff hurts." Finally, the anesthesiologists paralyzed all of his muscles with pancuronium just to wheel him to the surgical suite.

The operation was plagued with complications since it was performed under such suboptimal conditions. Now Mr. Goode lay in the recovery room, forty-eight hours post-op, on his way to losing the war with the microbes. The indefatigable bacteria had pillaged one organ after another, until each was substituted with a tube connected to an external machine.

The anesthesiologists and surgeons wanted him transferred out of the recovery room to the medical ICU. I had no desire to reacquire rights to this man, but forty-eight hours was the arbitrary statute of limitations for post-op complications. His medical problems could no longer be easily attributed to the surgery. They were simply his problems, and now they were ours. Reluctantly, I transferred him to our medical ICU. I left him with the ICU team, glad that I would not be the doctor caring for him.

Critically ill though he was, Mr. Goode somehow managed to improve. I'm not sure if it was his canny strength from life on the streets, or the fact that you just can't kill an old bully. But one by one, the tubes and catheters were gradually removed.

∽I lost track of Mr. Goode after that. Part of me is convinced that he is dead. If he wasn't killed in drug-related violence, he probably suffered repeated bouts of endocarditis until his heart valves simply withered away.

But maybe he'd managed to survive. For the years that I'd known him, his body had tolerated assaults that would have consumed another with a more ordinary constitution. Maybe his anger imbued his body with special strength. Maybe his war with the world gave him succor to live. Or maybe he was simply too nasty to die.

I'd never actually hated a patient before, but Harold Goode managed to squirrel right in under my skin. Having crossed paths at that critical juncture in my training when I was first in charge, Mr. Goode was able to hone right in on my insecurities and make me feel incompetent.

∽In considering becoming a doctor, I'd never imagined hating a patient. I suppose I assumed I'd like most of them, but truthfully I'd never even thought about the issue. Mr. Goode wrenched me from my naiveté. And why should hating a patient be unusual? After all, patients are just a subset of humanity. My interactions with Mr. Goode were so profoundly unsatisfying—how would I navigate my way with the inevitable patients of the future with whom I could not connect, or even respect? Could I be a good enough doctor for them? I wondered how much sacrifice I could make for a patient like Mr. Goode. Would I expend my reservoir of good will with the GI consult begging for an endoscopy for Mr. Goode? Would I skip lunch to wheel him to X-ray if he needed one right away? Would I give up a night of sleep tending to Mr. Goode if his oxygenation was dropping? The answer is, easily, yes. I didn't like Mr. Goode but of course I wanted him to live. I was, after all, a doctor in charge.

CHAPTER NINE

Time of Death: 3:27 A.M.

The day we die
the wind comes down
to take away
our footprints.

Song of the Southern Bushmen

THE PATIENT ARRIVED in the ER with a ruptured aorta from a car accident. The doctor jumped onto the stretcher and reached into the wound to grab the hemorrhaging vessel. Seconds later the patient was whisked off to surgery, with the doctor still straddling him upon the stretcher, clamping the aorta with his bare hand.

"Really, Rachel," I said, "this is ridiculous. This type of stuff doesn't happen in real life. First of all, he'd be wearing gloves. Second of all, no resident looks that attractive after twenty hours of working in the hospital."

The television show took place in an urban emergency room that was a bit reminiscent of Bellevue, except that the staff members were better coifed and had enough free time for multiple romantic involvements. There was definitely an air of realism, however, in the pace and the grittiness. It was entertaining and also gave my friends and family a taste of my life in the hospital.

When things were slow I would watch the show on the hospital TV. If my beeper was quiet I would telephone Rachel and provide live medical commentary on the action. It was our Thursday-night ritual.

ᐁ "Can you come see Mr. Teitelbaum?" A nurse's voice invaded my sleep. I was working overnight and had managed to fall asleep for a few hours. "He's just not looking so hot," she continued. "Could you just swing by and take a look?" Mumbling something in reply, I scraped my body out of bed, feet fumbling into my hospital clogs. I trudged over to the ward with the wooden clogs clomping, as it required too much energy to actually lift my feet off the ground.

Mr. Teitelbaum was an elderly gentleman sitting in a chair by the nurses' station—the spot always reserved for the slightly demented patients who'd "sundown" and become agitated at night. His hospital-issue pajamas drooped off his slight shoulders. A makeshift seatbelt constructed from a bedsheet pinned his frail body upright. His wizened face bobbed gently to the right.

As I approached him, one of the nurses tore off the bedsheet, yelling, "He's coding! He's coding! Call a code!" I got there just as they were tossing Mr. Teitelbaum onto a bed that had been wheeled into the hallway. He lay diagonally across the bed, a slip of a human body enmeshed in a heap of crisp white hospital sheets. "He's coding," the nurse yelled again.

The fatigue evaporated from my body with the sting of a plunge into ice water. "He's coding," echoed in my head—he's dying, right here in front of me. There were no other doctors around, just me. "He's coding,"—my mind froze onto that thought, unable to process what to do next. But luckily my body was able to react of its own accord and it leaped onto the bed and started doing CPR.

Elbows straight, fingers interlocked—press, release, press, release. Kneeling beside him, the weight of my whole body converged and was propelled from my shoulders through to my arms onto his body. I could feel his ancient chest giving way beneath me. Press, release, press, release.

"We can't do this in the hallway," the head nurse shouted. "There's no oxygen. Get him to his room!" With a jerk the bed began to move, with Mr. Teitelbaum lying askew on top of it and my body teetering precariously over Mr. Teitelbaum. Press, release, press, release. I pumped on his chest as the bed accelerated dizzily down the hallway.

"Code 411, Cardiac Arrest! 15-West!" blared the overhead speaker. "Code 411, 15-West!" A minute later, a crew of doctors arrived on 15-

West. They burst onto the ward just in time to get pelted with my clogs and stethoscope as the bed careened around a sharp corner. Press, release, press, release.

The bed skidded into Mr. Teitelbaum's room and slammed into the wall. The impact dislodged me from the bed and I catapulted forward, landing in the corner between the wall and the bed frame. Mr. Teitelbaum was immediately enveloped in a swarm of doctors and nurses. A burly intern hopped on the bed and took over my CPR role. I struggled to my feet and found myself pinned against the wall at the head of the bed. This was where the anesthesiologist normally stood in order to intubate, or put a breathing tube down the patient's trachea. I could see the anesthesiologist with her metal toolbox at the far end of the crowd, but I could not extricate myself from the sandwich of the bed and the wall and she could not negotiate the crowd to climb in.

Mr. Teitelbaum was being plunged in and out of the mattress as the intern thrust his bulk up and down upon the old man's chest. Another resident had flipped up Mr. Teitelbaum's gown and was starting to place a central line in the thigh. A third was prepping the electrical paddles. Two other residents were shouting out competing orders. Nurses were passing out meds. Medical students were crowding in to watch. The code was in full swing, except for one thing—Mr. Teitelbaum needed oxygen. He needed a breathing tube.

The anesthesiologist was trying in vain to wade through the frenetic crowd. She held her metal toolbox in front of her like a battering ram, but the noise and the bodies were impenetrable.

Time was of the essence. I had never intubated anyone before. As an internal medicine resident I'd only practiced on the plastic models in our CPR training course. And nobody's life was at stake there.

Should I try it? What if I failed? I could make things worse by wasting precious time and I would look like an utter idiot. A real code was not the time to be learning.

The bodies crowded around Mr. Teitelbaum, casting conflicting shadows over him. His body flopped in and out of the penumbra. Needles were going in, blood was coming out in tubes. Vials of epinephrine and atropine were discharging into his veins. He needed oxygen.

Would I waste more time by trying to climb out of my confinement? I could see the anesthesiologist elbowing at the throng. The medication cart and a beefy orderly blocked her path. I didn't have a choice.

"Intubation tray," I said firmly, holding out my hand to the nurse. The authority in my voice belied my terror. She handed me the equipment without hesitation. Didn't she know that I had no idea what I was doing? I mean, I'd played the "when in doubt, pretend" card before, but never in a code, and never in front of so many people.

I scrambled with the laryngoscope, clicking the pieces together as I'd seen the anesthesiologists do so many times. I hooked it in Mr. Teitelbaum's mouth to secure his jaw. Pull upward, not outward, I reminded myself. You don't want to break his teeth.

Break his teeth? The guy is almost dead. Forget about his teeth and get that tube in.

I pulled upward and outward trying to coax the epiglottis out of my line of sight so I could see into the trachea. His muscles and tissues lifted easily to my touch; I had thought there would be much more resistance. I leaned in closer, my nose practically inside Mr. Teitelbaum's mouth, and peered into his throat. The light of the laryngoscope shone down the tunnel.

There they were! There were landmark vocal cords joining in an upside-down V to mark the entrance to the trachea—the famous V that tells you that you've found your treasure. They glistened back at me, infinitely more beautiful than the rubber ones in the CPR models.

Okay, I told myself. This is it. Without diverting my eyes from the precious V of the vocal cords I shuffled my other hand in the mess of sheets until I'd located the plastic breathing tube. I took a deep breath and thrust the breathing tube between the cords. Obscuring my view as it entered, down it sailed into the depths of Mr. Teitelbaum.

Now the moment of truth. The most common mistake was to place the breathing tube into the more accessible esophagus. I prayed that the tube had made it safely through the V and hadn't veered off course. If it ended up in the esophagus, I'd be humiliated in front of all these doctors and nurses. And Mr. Teitelbaum wouldn't be doing much better, what with all that precious oxygen piling into his stomach instead of his lungs.

Since the very act of placing the breathing tube automatically blocked one's view, there was no way to know where it had ended up until one listened with a stethoscope to the stomach and then the lungs. The former should be silent and the latter should be brimming with breath sounds.

The respiratory technician pumped oxygen into the tube now sticking out of Mr. Teitelbaum's mouth. Please, please, let that oxygen be sailing down the trachea, not the esophagus, I whispered. The anesthesiologist had finally elbowed her way to the bedside. She placed her stethoscope onto Mr. Teitelbaum's stomach and listened carefully. She held up her hand to transiently halt CPR so she could hear. She slid the bell of her stethoscope to the left lung, and then to the right, and then to the stomach. The entire crowd was silent, their eyes following the trail of her stethoscope. I was too afraid to breathe.

She shrugged. "It's in," she said blandly. Her body was already halfway out the door. The breathing tube was in—her job was over.

I sank back against the wall in my tiny confinement and my head slumped forward against the bed frame. It's in, it's in, I panted deliriously to myself. I wiped off the perspiration that had collected along the rim of my eyebrows. It's in!

I took an extra fraction of a second to bask in my private glory—no one else had known that it was my first time. I had just done something dramatic and definitive to save someone's life. I'd never done that before. It was like the way Zalman Wiszhinsky had been saved with the needle in his chest to remove the fluid around his heart. I suddenly felt the immense distance from when I was that third-year medical student who was so confused and lost watching Mr. Wiszhinsky's pericardiocentisis to the resident I was now, who'd just made a split-second decision that might save someone's life. It was only a few years, but my fingers and my brain had now grown comfortable doing things that I never could have imagined before. I was really feeling like a doctor.

But there was still a code going on and I didn't have the luxury of much philosophizing. I gathered myself off the floor and joined the action with my colleagues. In seconds I was fully engrossed in the energy of the code—injecting medications, delivering electric shocks, drawing blood. Vials of epinephrine and 4x4 gauze pads sailed back and forth. This one shouted at that one in the chain of command. The acrid smell of burnt skin and chest hairs rose from the electric paddles. But my eyes kept snapping back to that plastic tube that was delivering oxygen to Mr. Teitelbaum's lungs.

"Thank you very much, everybody." Sudden silence.

Those universal code-ending words rang out at 3:27 A.M. Mr. Teitelbaum was officially dead; my breathing tube had been futile. Someone said he'd had several heart attacks and strokes in the past. He was ninety-one years old and severely demented. On this night a malignant arrhythmia had hijacked his heart.

The crowd dissipated and the nurse's aides remained to clean him up. They pulled out the central line. They removed the EKG electrodes. And then they pulled out my breathing tube. I watched it exit his lungs, traveling on the reverse course that I had so nervously dispatched it only twenty minutes ago. My life-saving tube was dumped in the garbage along with all the other unnecessary equipment. There was a catch in my stomach. One of the aides yanked the curtain around Mr. Teitelbaum to start the process of cleaning. The beige and yellow-striped cloth slashed a boundary between me and Mr. Teitelbaum and I was now on the outside.

I left the room, suddenly feeling lonely. Lonely for Mr. Teitelbaum, who'd died all alone, despite the breathing tube that I'd agonized over. Despite the breathing tube that had signified such a landmark in my training as a doctor—it was the first time I'd "saved" a life. Or was it? Was a breathing tube any more a life-saver than the blood pressure medicine I'd given last week in clinic to Mrs. Hernandez or the flu shot I'd finally convinced Mr. Leung to get? My feet felt slippery on the linoleum and I looked down to discover that I was wearing only socks. There were brown splotches on them from iodine that had splattered during the code. I shuffled down the hallway, the end of each step slipping nearly out of control from the overwaxed floors. There in the far corner was one of my wayward clogs. Two rooms down was the other. I slid them on, my feet sinking into the familiar indentations. Where was my stethoscope? It had flown off when we'd rounded the corner. I hunted up and down the hallway until I finally found it snagged around one of the railings.

I settled down in the nurses' station with Mr. Teitelbaum's chart. Since Mr. Teitelbaum was a patient of one of the residents who I was covering overnight, it was my responsibility to document the code. I opened the chart gingerly, dreading the unending morass of papers that typically accompanies elderly, chronically ill patients. The thought of sifting through tangles of illegible notes chronicling one illness after another wearied me before I could even begin.

But I opened the cover and there was nothing. Nothing at all. I found myself face to face with the nakedness of an empty chart. Mr. Teitelbaum, it turned out, had only been admitted to the hospital a few hours ago. The progress notes were entirely blank—he hadn't had time to progress.

And so I entered the very first progress note in Leo Teitelbaum's chart, entitled "Expiration Note." I printed neatly, self conscious that mine would be the only note in the official record of his sojourn at our hospital. The story of the man who's life I'd saved who didn't actually live.

> Called by RNs to evaluate patient. Patient unresponsive without pulse. CPR begun. Patient intubated (!). EKG revealed v-tach. Defibrillation x 4 without success. Rhythm degenerated to v-fib then asystole. Unresponsive to epinephrine and atropine. No palpable blood pressure. Code terminated after 20 minutes. Time of death: 3:27 a.m.

I reread the note, abashed by its brevity. A human being had ended ninety-one years of life and these disembodied words constituted the official record. Mr. Teitelbaum had died without any family members around him. Just a group of strangers on the midnight shift.

I sat back in my chair, wondering about Leo Teitelbaum. I supposed he was born somewhere in Eastern Europe. Was he from a small town like Zalman Wiszhinsky? Did he escape murderous thugs by sneaking through the forest, or did he board a luxury ocean liner to come to America? Did he come through Ellis Island like my grandfather Irving? Had his English ever lost its accent? Did he drink tea with a sugar cube in his mouth? I would never know.

I apologized for being a stranger. For accompanying him through this intimate rite without ever knowing how his voice sounded or what his touch was like. I apologized for all the pain and chaos we had put him through during his final moments. I wished he'd had a quieter ending like Elba Rodriguez, rectal exam notwithstanding. And I thanked him for the opportunity to test a skill I wasn't sure I possessed, even if it didn't do him any good in the end. Mr. Teitelbaum gave me the confidence to know that I could do it if such a situation ever arose again.

My memory of Leo Teitelbaum would be only of this night. Of zooming down the hall on a speeding bed, pounding on his frail little chest with my shoes flying off. Of the personal moment of truth as I drove the breathing tube down his throat. Of the surprisingly little resistance his body offered. Of the "unsuccessful" code. Of the 3:27 A.M. time of death. Of the 3:30 A.M. phone call to his family. Of falling back to sleep at four A.M. Of calling Rachel the next morning to share my experience.

"Really Rachel, I was flying down the hall on the stretcher ..."

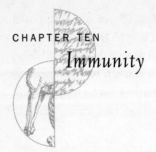

CHAPTER TEN

Immunity

HER TEETH SEEMED ENORMOUS, but that was only because the rest of her face had receded so. The flesh had ebbed back, shrinking from contoured fullness to spare, arid outlines. Fragile porcelain skin lay draped over the angular bones, like sheets over spindly furniture. Translucent freckles dotted the landscape, but weren't enough to impart color. Her hair was brittle and red, with furtive spots of scalp peering through. In places, the amber hues had faded to a waxen yellow. But her eyes were blue, disarmingly blue, the heavy ocean blue of youthful eyes—eyes not old enough for cataracts or glaucoma to cloud them.

From my vantage point ten feet away, I indulged in my one minute Bellevue analysis. Diagnosis: end-stage AIDS. Current illness: Disseminated cryptococcus or lymphoma. Prognosis: two to three weeks. Treatment priority: get that DNR signed.

The rapidity of my assessment startled me. Somewhere along the way during the middle of residency, I had started to develop that elusive quality I'd been longing for: clinical instinct. When had it arisen? I couldn't point to any one time, but I realized that I now doubted myself a bit less than before. And I couldn't deny the effect of experience—at this point I'd cared for so many AIDS patients, including two months on the designated AIDS ward. AIDS wasn't so frightening anymore; it was just a disease like any other. I was vigilant with needles, but no more so than with other patients, since I never knew who might be harboring unknown AIDS or hepatitis or any other virus.

The feeling of clinical instinct was like a thirst being gently slaked, without the utilitarian necessity of water. The relief of knowledge making itself known without agony. This young woman had AIDS. She was end-stage and needed a DNR. I didn't yet know the immediate illness that brought her in today, but I felt relatively clear about her underlying disease. I had a road map—a familiar road map—and I felt prepared to set out on the journey.

Two middle-aged women materialized from behind the curtain. They wore sensible polyester outfits with orthopedic shoes and gripped their purses tightly to their bodies. The taller one had faded gray hair puffed in a 1950s style. Sharp lipstick covered her thin, tight lips. Heavy furrows were hewn in her cheeks, which were bare of any other makeup.

She reached for my forearm. Her voice was flat and deliberate. "She's going to be okay, isn't she? You're going to make Eileen better, right?"

Make her better? The incongruity of the skeleton on the stretcher and the innocent optimism of the question stunned me into silence.

She continued talking before I could even begin to formulate any words to bridge that chilling gap between our respective interpretations of reality. "I'm Mrs. O'Neil, her mother. This," she said, pointing with her purse, "is Eileen's aunt." The aunt was half a head shorter and wider-set at the hips. Thin wisps of gray and white hair were cut in a nondescript bob around her head. Her face looked worn and haggard like her sister's, but her wrinkles softened as she smiled at me. A twinkle eased its way out of the pale blue of her eyes, which were tinged with flecks of opacity.

I turned back toward Eileen, who was staring blankly at the ceiling. Her face seemed to have no muscles left with which to create any facial expression. There were only the chafing bony girders of her skull, and the craters in which floated those unearthly blue eyes. I rested my palms on the rail of the stretcher and leaned in toward her. "Eileen," I asked, "how long have you been feeling ill?" There was no response.

Mrs. O'Neil jumped in. "Not too long now. I guess a few weeks. Is that right?" Her sister nodded in agreement, her cropped hair moving as one with her head. I asked them to tell me about Eileen's illness.

The mother shrugged her shoulders. "Nothing much, I guess. Just not feeling like herself the last little while."

"Has Eileen ever been sick before?"

"No. She's always been a healthy one, all of her thirty-five years. A hard worker always." Mrs. O'Neil paused. "It's really only been these last few weeks that she's been a bit under the weather. More tired, I guess."

I turned back to Eileen. "How are you feeling, Eileen?" Again, no response.

Mrs. O'Neil whispered to me, "She has some trouble with her hearing, you know. You have to speak loudly."

I shouted my question in Eileen's ear. Slowly, those vivid blue eyes wobbled toward me. Her parched lips struggled with the air. She parsed her words in a hoarse whisper, gasping with each syllable. "Take … me … home. I … feel … fine." Faint stirrings emanated from her emaciated body. The wispy muscles of her shoulders began to quiver. I assumed she was rearranging herself on the stretcher for a more comfortable position. But her gaunt fingers crept forward, scaling the metal railing with an odd alchemy of aching effort and eerie weightlessness. The pads of her fingers ratcheted up the silvery pole in fits and starts—stalling at patches of friction then wincing several millimeters forward on serendipitous momentum. I realized that she was attempting to sit herself up, to provide action to bolster her demand to be taken home. But the guardrail consisted of two bars and her hand had depleted itself by the first. It remained stranded there for several moments, spindly bird claws quivering to encircle a branch, until its grip gave out and it collapsed in upon itself, crumpling onto the bedsheet.

It was clear that I couldn't take a history from Eileen. I led the mother and the aunt a few steps aside to get some information. I started in a low voice, but Mrs. O'Neil waved my precautions away. "Don't worry," she said, "Eileen can't hear you. If you don't shout good and loud, it's like you're not even there. Besides, Eileen's always been the dreamy type, even as a little one, always off in her own dreamworld. She won't pay you no mind."

"Where does Eileen live?" I asked.

"At home," she replied, with a touch of surprise in her voice. "We're a family—me, her, the boys. Three generations under one roof, right here on First Avenue." She smiled and turned to Eileen's aunt. "And with my sister just around the corner we're a regular Irish clan."

Eileen's boys?

"Peter, he's at the Sacred Heart grammar school, and Tommy, he's almost graduated now. One more year at boarding school." She smiled wistfully. "He's so big now. Getting to be a real man." Her sister smiled and nodded with her.

The father?

"He's not here," she said. Her gaze focused away from mine ever so slightly.

Her job?

"Eileen is very active in the church. She works at the Sunday school."

A teacher?

Mrs. O'Neil paused. "Well, no, not exactly. She helps out with the materials and stuff. And she loves kids. And the church. She's always volunteering for the bake sales. She never misses Mass."

Who is supporting the boys?

Mrs. O'Neil took a short, tight breath. "I have my Social Security and pension. It's not always easy, but ..." She looked straight at me and I could see the brown speckles within the faded blue of her eyes. "We are an Irish family, doctor; we take care of our own. No one should ever want for nothing in a family." Her sister nodded somberly.

I asked more about the father of the boys. The two women looked at each other and then Mrs. O'Neil sighed. "That was all a long time ago, doctor. Now we are all a family and take care of each other."

Has she had any other boyfriends?

Mrs. O'Neil drew back. "Oh, no! Eileen would never do that. She's Catholic."

Did she ever smoke, drink, or take any drugs? Mrs. O'Neil shook her head firmly. "Eileen has lived with me ever since she was born. The church is the most important thing in her life. She has never done anything like that. That much I know."

I left them and went to examine Eileen. She lay immobile on the stretcher while I listened to her lungs and shone my penlight in her eyes. She lay passive as I poked at her liver and prodded her spleen. It was almost as though I was examining a patient in a coma. Except for those crystal blue eyes that floated languidly about the room. Every so often they would catch mine, lock mine in a brief embrace. I imagined they were trying to talk to me, to tell me what was going on inside of her eroded shell. But the effort was too much and they'd disengage to continue their aimless roaming.

Surprisingly, I found no telltale signs of AIDS. Or of any other particular illness, for that matter. Her lungs were clear, her abdomen was soft. She had no signs of meningitis or pneumonia, no evidence of an abscess anywhere. She had no oral thrush, no swollen lymph nodes, no rash. Her blood tests were relatively normal and her chest X-ray was clear. Maybe my road map was not as clear as I had assumed.

Aside from a fever of 103 degrees, I could not find any other objective abnormalities. There was no physical sign, laboratory abnormality, or symptom that I could latch onto to make a specific diagnosis. She was just emaciated.

Clearly this illness had been progressing for far longer than the few weeks her family admitted to. Eileen had bedsores and signs of skin breakdown. She weighed less than ninety pounds. At this point it almost didn't matter what particular disease she had. Whatever it was, it was near the end. That I had certainly learned in my time at Bellevue.

I led the mother and the aunt to the storage area—the quietest place I could find in the ER. These "family talks" were always the worst. My mouth yearned to deliver words of optimism, of treatment plans, of convalescence and recovery. How joyful and nearly instinctive was the lexicon of success rates and outpatient follow-up visits and preventative medical care. My soul squirmed when that vocabulary was denied. All that was left was a rasping emptiness, a void into which I had to contort to create words to render the horrible palatable.

In theory, it sounded so simple. Be straightforward and honest with your patients, we'd been told by our attendings and our society.

Straightforward and honest. "Your daughter is going to die." So easy on paper, so obvious in clinical discussions on rounds. But entirely un-pronounceable to human beings standing on the ground before you—human beings staring at you with eyes blinking in slow-motion be-wilderment, lips furrowed and parched from nervous teeth-biting, skin tightening around the face as twenty-odd muscles quivered with the strain of controlling emotions. How can you look at the souls with whom you are sharing breaths in the eighteen intimate inches of oxy-gen between you and say, "Your daughter is going to die." How is that humanly possible?

The three of us cramped ourselves between the cases of IV saline and the stacks of chest tube trays. "I don't know exactly what is wrong with Eileen," I started. *Of course I know what's wrong with her—I'm still sure it's AIDS—but I can't get the damn words out,* my logical mind railed at me. "I can't say for sure what's going on, but whatever it is . . . whatever it is, it is probably very serious." *Stop beating around the bush. Just say what you know is true. You know she is near death.* "I think she has been sick for a while." *Is that the best you can do?*

The two women nodded methodically, with preternatural calm. *Come on, don't avoid the real issue. You have to tell them what the situa-tion is.* I hesitated and lowered my voice. "If her sons want to be with her, now is probably the time." They continued to nod.

How can you expect your patients to be strong if you are such a weak-ling? Don't sneak out without facing the hard stuff. Don't get into the de-nial game. I took a deep breath to quell my own stomach and then blurted out, "I am concerned that she might have AIDS." *Okay, you did it. You got it on the table.* I waited for a reaction, but they did not flinch. They stood rock solid in the swirl of the ER chaos, clasping their purses, nodding their heads stoically.

The aunt took my hand. "Tommy, he's the big boy. He's leaving for boarding school in two days. Maybe he shouldn't go?"

I bit hard on the edge of my tongue, sending lancing pains shooting through to my gums. How could I answer this question with certainty? How could I take away hope, but how could I not warn them of possible impending death? How could I live with myself if Eileen's children missed their only chance to say good-bye?

"I think..." I said gingerly. "I think maybe you should have him come in tomorrow." I curled my stinging tongue inward, hoping I wasn't erring on the wrong side. "There might not be much time." They nodded at me. I peered at their faces, trying to read a reaction in their heavy wrinkles. But their mechanical nodding and granite stares refused to allow me to judge the impact of my words. Had they absorbed anything I'd said?

I watched Mrs. O'Neil and her sister as they walked out of the ER arm in arm, their purses firmly secured against their bodies. Their orthopedic shoes paced in rhythm. I wished the ER were not such a noisy, smelly, horrible place.

I trudged back to the main area of the emergency room where Eileen O'Neil lay limp on the stretcher. What was I going to do with her? What specific infection or illness should I treat her for? Although I felt that AIDS was the most likely cause of her overall condition, I had, in fact, no hard evidence.

Alone with Eileen I asked her again about various AIDS risk factors. With feeble shakes of her head, she denied them all. I asked her specific questions about her sexual history. In a strained whisper she told me that she'd had sex only twice in her life, both times with the same man and that's how she'd had her two sons. I rephrased the question as many ways as I could, but she resolutely denied ever having sexual intercourse outside of those two instances. And she didn't want an HIV test.

Despite the lack of information, I had to come up with a treatment plan. What to treat her for? Even if she did have AIDS, which I could not prove, what was the specific illness that was plaguing her right now? The admission form had a blank for "admitting diagnosis" that I was required to fill in. The order sheet demanded names of medications and dosages and frequencies of administration. The reality of medical care did not permit me the luxury of dwelling in the nonspecific. I had to choose a diagnosis and implement a treatment plan.

I reviewed the history, physical exam, and lab values again. There was no clue, no tip-off to the immediate problem. I thought about "watchful waiting," as I'd done with Harold Goode—sitting still until the disease declared itself and only then institute treatment. But unlike Mr. Goode, with his hefty muscles and imposing bulk, Eileen O'Neil didn't look as if she could make it through the night on observation alone.

I would have to treat her empirically, but what to treat? Any medication I chose would have side effects, potentially toxic. I could even kill her with my treatments. I chewed on the edge of my Styrofoam coffee cup, pressing uneven scalloped designs along the edge. What infections might kill her tonight? What could I absolutely not afford to miss?

I asked Eileen again if she would agree to an HIV test. With a limp quaver, she shook her head no.

An open bag of potato chips was sitting on the clerk's desk. It had probably been there since the last shift, but I plowed through them anyway. I decided to treat Eileen for pneumocystis pneumonia. PCP was the most common pneumonia in AIDS, so the statistics were on my side, despite the fact that Eileen wasn't coughing or short of breath, and that her chest X-ray was clear. But without treatment, PCP could kill rapidly. And luckily, PCP could be successfully treated with antibiotics. It was one of the few HIV-related infections that could possibly be cured. Practically the only one. If I had to gamble, this was one of the few bets that might pay off. I felt that slight tinge of warmth again around my neck—clinical instinct. An odd but gratifying sensation. Something just felt right to me. I couldn't say why it felt right, but it did.

It wasn't a very satisfying diagnosis or treatment plan, however, because I didn't have any evidence for my decision, but I couldn't think of anything else to do for her. The high dose of Bactrim, though potentially toxic to her kidneys in her malnourished state, would also treat regular pneumonia and any possible urinary tract infections.

I was already out the door, walking home through the Bellevue garden, when I spun around and stormed back in. I grabbed Eileen's chart and scribbled an order for an additional antibiotic. "Double coverage," my instinct told me. Maybe I'd sleep better that night.

First Avenue was deserted at that time of night. I walked along the edge of the empty sidewalk unable to shake the image of Eileen's cadaverous body and skeletal face. Where did Eileen come from? How did she just appear at the end stages of her illness? My stomach was curdling from the potato chips and coffee.

Eileen and her family insisted that she'd only been ill for a few weeks. That was impossible! She had obviously been seriously ill for many months but nobody had ever sought medical attention. Didn't anyone notice that she had withered away to eighty-seven pounds? Was nobody alarmed that she barely had the strength to talk?

The chilly October night air needled through my thin white coat. I wished I'd worn a real jacket. Eileen's mother and aunt seemed like responsible, hardworking women. Why didn't they do anything? And Eileen, she was thirty-five years old! Why didn't she seek help for herself as she grew weaker and weaker? Was there a conspiracy to hide this illness, or was everyone in such complete denial that they'd never even noticed it? Was Eileen invisible in her own family?

I got home and poured myself some milk of magnesia. The chalky lemon-mint flavor was revolting and not the least bit reassuring. How could anyone not notice a person dying in their midst?

✑The next day, Sunday, was our "short day." The plan was to round on our patients, present the new admissions to the attending, and be out by noon to enjoy the autumn weekend. Based on her location, Eileen would be the last patient to be seen on rounds, so I decided to take a quick peek at her before formal rounds began. I walked in sipping my coffee and trying to get a bite of my bagel, to see Eileen heaving with violent convulsions. The nurses hadn't yet made it to her bedside.

I tossed my coffee and bagel into the garbage and ran to her bed feeling my own breathing tighten. What had happened? Was she dying already? Eileen's eyes had rolled back and her body was twitching. It was clear that she was having a grand mal seizure. I could practically hear the bones of her skeletal body rattling from the seizure as they hiccuped and jostled off the bed. "Valium, ten milligrams, *stat*," I called out, before I even could formulate the thought. The nurse had the vial in my hands almost before the words had exited my mouth. Eileen writhed and jerked as I maneuvered the needle into the vial as quickly as possible without pricking my own fingers with it. I drew up the ten milligrams then discharged it into her IV. Like a wave of tranquility whispering over her, the Valium slowly eased her shuddering. Gradually the tension in her muscles softened and Eileen sank into a drowsy post-seizure state. And my body relaxed in kind, as though the Valium had trickled backward through her vein to the IV, into the syringe, through to my hand, and over my body.

I sat next to her bed and watched her for the next thirty minutes to make sure she was still breathing. I'd told my interns to do rounds without me. In my hand I held a syringe with Dilantin, an antiseizure medication that was longer acting than Valium. Every few minutes I injected a bit more, watching the cardiac monitor overhead for any possible arrhythmias from the large loading dose of the drug.

When I was convinced that she was reasonably stable—no further seizures, no cardiac abnormalities, no breathing problems—I dragged her stretcher up to the third floor for a stat CT scan of her head. No transport services on weekends.

The radiology hallway was deserted. Eileen was asleep from the Valium and I sat on the floor next to her stretcher waiting for the CT technician to call us. Signs overhead pointed patients toward X-ray, Ultrasound, Mammogram, and Nuclear Medicine. Directions were in English, Spanish, and Chinese. Without actual patients here to follow these directions, though, they suddenly seemed so bereft and incongruous, like traffic cops without any traffic. I leaned back against the wall.

Sundays at Bellevue were quiet affairs—silent hallways, empty elevators, hollow spaces. Not quite as lonely as night-float, because at least there was sunlight in the patients' rooms that lined the outer perimeter of the building, but certainly solitary. From where I was sitting on the floor, I couldn't see Eileen's body on the stretcher, just the metal framework and wheels parked on an angle. I suddenly realized how hungry I was and wished I hadn't thrown away my coffee and bagel.

When it was our turn, I maneuvered the stretcher into the room around the bulky CT machine with its looming metal doughnut. I helped the technician lift Eileen out of the stretcher onto the table. Her body was so light and motionless, it was as though we were lifting a lifeless mannequin. Three times I checked her pulse and breathing to make sure she was alive. Faint, but still present.

The technician assured me that the films would make their way to the radiologist, but I knew how things usually went on a Sunday and I told him that I would wait for them myself. Another twenty silent minutes in the empty hallway staring at the signs and finally the films were printed. I dragged Eileen's stretcher back to the elevator with the films crammed under my arm. I walked the films to the radiologist on the first floor and waited while he scanned the forty images of Eileen's brain sliced every which way. He pronounced it "normal." "Normal," he added dryly, "for a ninety-year-old." Her cortex resembled a shrunken apple, with yawning gaps between the folds of tissue. The shriveled pleats of white matter seemed stranded, isolated islands in vast seas of black emptiness. There was no doubt that Eileen had been sick for a very long time. But aside from the atrophy, there were no focal abnormalities to explain a seizure: no abscess, no tumor, no classic AIDS infections.

Resigning myself to losing my Sunday entirely, I prepped Eileen for a spinal tap. The interns were still off doing their scut, but Kim and Francois, the medical students, had wandered down to join me. I showed them how I prepped Eileen's back with iodine and sterile drapes. I anesthetized the area where I planned to insert the spinal needle. Eileen was so gaunt that the needle slipped effortlessly between her vertebrae.

The needle slid through Eileen's paper-thin skin, with hardly any underlying tissue to impede its passage. The needle had barely gone beneath the surface when the cerebrospinal flowed out. I collected the precious droplets in my tubes while Kim and Francois looked on. I thought about this fluid swimming through the cavernous spaces within Eileen's skull, the expanded reservoirs left behind as her brain had withered away. I stored the tubes in my pocket as I trundled with the students through the maze of laboratories on the fourth floor, hand-delivering each one to the respective chemistry, hematology, cytology, and microbiology labs.

The results showed no suggestions of meningitis. Her blood tests were similarly unrevealing. Eileen was so sick, yet I could not find any signs of a specific illness. I felt like I was in a twilight zone with her. She and her family were convinced that she wasn't sick and there was nothing telltale to distinguish exactly what was making her sick, yet she was nearly wasted away to death.

Meanwhile, her blood pressure had been slipping downward. Not so much so to start panicking, but low enough to begin administering large volumes of IV fluids. Because she was so emaciated and had so few veins accessible I decided to place a central line in her neck. If nothing else, this Sunday was turning out to be a great day to teach the students how to do all these procedures.

"The clavicle is your landmark for a subclavian central line," I said to Kim and Francois as I sterilized Eileen's skin. Her clavicle jutted out from her chest in prominent bas-relief. There was no fat or muscle to obscure its definition. "Insert your needle and advance it until you hit the bone." I pushed my needle forward and it immediately stopped short against Eileen's protuberant clavicle. "Now comes the tricky part, getting the needle under the bone. Push your needle downward, but not too much downward because there's a lot of lung sitting under there. There's no better way to ruin a Sunday than by collapsing a lung." Nervous laughter from the students

I eased my needle below Eileen's clavicle. Kim and Francois leaned in to see. Their eager puppy faces, panting to see yet another exciting medical procedure, crowded into the work area, but I didn't mind. "Now once you're under the bone," I said, "you turn the needle inward and point toward the trachea. Start advancing it slowly, aiming toward the midline of the body. But not too far; you don't want to puncture the trachea." More nervous laughter. I hadn't gone more than two millimeters when blood suddenly flashed into the syringe. My heart sparkled.

No matter how dire or depressing a patient's situation is, it can never take away that momentary delicious feeling of blood flashing into the syringe. Eileen's gauntness had been my bonus because there was barely any meat for the needle to travel through. This was probably the easiest subclavian line I'd ever done. But as soon as I'd enjoyed my fleeting moment of pleasure—heightened, of course, by having done it in front of a group of awestruck medical students—the reality of the situation and the very reason why I was even putting in a central line flooded right back at me. After the bravado of slipping in the central line on the first try and suturing neat one-handed stitches, I was still left with an emaciated woman not much older than I who was about to die from something that I couldn't quite figure out, much less do anything about.

Between procedures, I discussed the case by phone with Dr. Liang, my attending. He disagreed with my working diagnosis of AIDS. He was concerned that she had cancer hidden somewhere in her body. Dr. Liang's suggestion was to undertake a thorough search for a malignancy that would include CT scans of her chest, abdomen, and pelvis, a mammogram, a bone marrow biopsy, a bone scan, and maybe even taking her up the block to NYU for an MRI. We didn't have an MRI at Bellevue then. I spent what was left of Sunday filling out forms and making telephone calls to arrange these tests.

Eileen O'Neil had snatched up what could have been my last autumn weekend to enjoy the outdoors. I tramped home in the heavy shadows of the Bellevue parking garage where the concrete chill pervaded the street. Turning the corner, though, I spotted a rapidly fading bit of light on Twenty-ninth Street where a low-slung deli on Second Avenue allowed a sliver to come through. The sun wasn't all gone yet! I dashed over to the spot and found an old crate that was probably the regular roost of one of the homeless guys from the Bellevue Men's Shelter. I positioned it up against a brick wall, angling it to take maximum advantage of this commodity that was so gingerly rationed by the city's skyscrapers. I planted myself in that evanescent patch of summer. I basked in ten whole minutes of delicious sunshine before it disintegrated below the skyline.

Residency wasn't so bad after all.

&The next day Eileen's blood pressure remained low despite the fluids infusing through my beautifully placed central line with my tidy one-handed stitches. I decided to transfer Eileen to the ICU for closer monitoring. She still refused an HIV test and I still had no diagnosis. Maybe my clinical instinct wasn't correct, after all. Sitting at the nurses' station reviewing the case with my colleagues who would be taking over her care, I caught sight of Eileen on the closed-circuit monitor. Her mother was sitting beside her trying to feed her lunch brought from home. When Mrs. O'Neil held a spoon to her mouth, Eileen raised her skeletal arm and fought her off. The mother tried again and again. Each time, Eileen managed to muster the strength to physically push her mother away. This continued for nearly thirty minutes.

Mrs. O'Neil passed me on her way out, her purse clasped in one hand, the plastic containers of food in the other. She smiled at me and said brightly, "We did well today. She ate almost everything I brought." As she walked away I could see that the containers were entirely full.

Dr. Redlin, the ICU attending, disagreed with my presumptive diagnosis of HIV. So much so that he insisted on stopping the Bactrim. "You have no evidence to support PCP," he said. "Her chest X-ray is clear, her oxygen saturation is normal, she's not coughing. She's not even vaguely short of breath! You are going to ruin her kidneys with this high antibiotic dose." The next morning was our weekly case management conference for the entire medical housestaff. Our team was chosen to present Eileen's case to a guest attending for its "diagnostic challenges." Dr. Connelly also did not think that it was AIDS. He felt that she might be suffering from a hidden cancer or perhaps anorexia nervosa.

I was feeling more confused and more in doubt about my clinical instinct. Perhaps I wasn't ready yet to make a one-minute diagnosis, but still, nothing else made sense. Anorexia usually occurs in teenagers, but Eileen was thirty-five. Cancer was a possibility, but we had CTed every inch of her emaciated body and could find nothing. It seemed like all the attendings were determined to find any diagnosis other than HIV in this white, Catholic woman. Perhaps I was biased, but young people who looked like concentration camp victims in New York City in the early 1990s usually had AIDS. Unless she had a rare genetic syndrome or some exotic tropical disease. But it was the attendings who always admonished the medical students—"When you hear hoofbeats, look for horses, not zebras."

✑Eileen stabilized in the ICU and was transferred back to my team a few days later. I learned from her family that Eileen had been sick for at least a few months, and that despite her mother's pleadings, would not see a doctor. She had grown so weak that she could no longer get up from the living room couch. One day the priest from her church had paid a visit. He was horrified to see how wasted she'd become and, ignoring her protests, had dialed 911. When the ambulance arrived, Eileen was simply too weak to refuse.

I questioned Eileen about her health in the past year. She answered all of my questions with a monotonous, saccharine tone accompanied by her gaunt toothy smile. Even when I asked difficult or embarrassing questions, she used the same cloyingly sweet voice. She didn't always hear, or appear to understand, what was asked. The lapses, though, were not consistent. But she definitely did not want an HIV test. I began to wonder if there was an element of developmental delay or emotional handicap. Something was just not right.

Later on that week we had our monthly "professor rounds." This was a special session with Dr. Malawi, one of the most respected attendings. It was a treat to have the undivided attention of a senior attending for two hours and the luxury to delve into a single case.

We chose to present the case of Eileen O'Neil, who had been with us for two weeks now without any diagnosis. We brought Dr. Malawi to her bedside, where he questioned her gently but extensively. His physical exam was thorough; he palpated her spleen, percussed her diaphragm, inspected her fingernail beds, and examined her retinas. Together we combed through the data. Dr. Malawi ran his fingers through his trim white beard as we reviewed all the labs in exhaustive detail and examined every single X-ray and CT scan. For two hours we probed every detail of Eileen's case.

Dr. Malawi felt that the clinical picture was most consistent with anorexia nervosa, and that we were seeing the nonspecific end stages of profound starvation. He distinctly did not think it was HIV.

Sitting in our tiny doctors' station, my frustration was beginning to boil. This was the fourth attending who thought I was completely wrong in my diagnosis. I was starting to doubt my own reality. "But what about the seizure?" I asked. I had witnessed her body convulsing furiously; it had been real. "And her atrophied brain?"

Dr. Malawi shook his head. "They were probably both due to the severe malnutrition and associated metabolic abnormalities. Beside, she doesn't have any risk factors for AIDS."

My patience broke. "She's had two children—that's two risk factors!"

Was there a generation gap, I wondered, or was I overestimating my clinical acumen? Four senior doctors thought I was wrong and that I had given her improper and toxic medications on her first night. I ground my teeth, hoping that my beeper would go off so I could escape from this humiliating conference. But it didn't and I had to sit through the full two hours nursing my anger.

I was still fuming the next morning when I ran into my intern by the elevator. SaraBeth looked more haggard than the usual intern fatigue. She told me that she had not gone home the previous night, that she had ended up spending the entire night in the hospital.

"After you went home," she explained in her insufferably slow Southern drawl, "the nurses called me to see Eileen." SaraBeth paused for a long breath. "They said she was short of breath." Another pause.

"Yes?" I asked, unable to mask the tinge of annoyance in my voice.

SaraBeth continued in her methodical monotone. "When I examined her, I couldn't really hear any breath sounds on the left side." Silence.

I waved my hands in the air. "And so . . . ?"

"Weeeelll . . . I ordered a chest X-ray." More silence.

"And . . . ?" I was ready to choke her.

"Well they—the radiologists—said her whole left lung had collapsed."

"What?" I said, snapping out of my impatience. "She had a pneumothorax? What happened? Did you put in another central line without telling me?"

"No." She paused to tuck some loose hair behind her ear. "The lung collapsed all by itself, it seems. It was a spontaneous pneumothorax." She articulated each syllable as though she were reading a story to preschoolers.

"A spontaneous pneumothorax?" I grabbed at her shoulders. "A spontaneous pneumo? Why didn't you call me at home?"

SaraBeth looked at me with a confused expression, trying to figure out what I was driving at. "She's doing much better now," she offered tentatively. "I called the cardiovascular surgeons right away." Her timid eyes faltered and her voice slowed even more. "They put in a chest tube to re-expand her lung."

"Do you know what a spontaneous pneumothorax means?" My tired intern blinked at me without speaking. I guess she was waiting for me to berate her for something she'd done wrong. "Do you understand what this means?" Anger and frustration that had been building up over the past two weeks finally erupted and I practically shouted as I shook her by the shoulders and wrung out that excruciating Southern charm. "She has PCP!"

I restarted the Bactrim. Two days later the HIV test came back positive.

✑I have always dreaded breaking the news of AIDS, but here I felt truly overwhelmed. There were so many complicating factors in this particular case, so I sought assistance from the HIV counselor. Mary Lou was one of my favorite people at Bellevue, known for generously dispensing good humor, sound advice, and free condoms in equal measure. A full shock of white hair spilled over her crinkled eyes and pink-rimmed glasses. A necklace of keys jounced and jingled over her trademark corduroy overalls. Her energy and enthusiasm were more than I had seen in most people in their thirties, much less in their sixties.

Together we sat down at Eileen's bedside. Mary Lou began by reviewing with Eileen the basics about the HIV test. She hadn't gotten past the definition of "antibody" when I noticed that Eileen's eyes were starting to moisten. Tentative drops unfolded over her lashes. Mary Lou was talking about the meaning of false positives and false negatives. The tears piled up and gathered momentum at the edges of her eyelids. Mary Lou explained the use of the initial ELISA test versus the confirmatory Western blot assay. A few droplets escaped from the enlarging crescent of liquid and began to dribble down the hollow of Eileen's cheekbones. Before Mary Lou could even get to the specifics of Eileen's test, a deluge of tears burst forth. Months of powerful denial came crashing down. Eileen sobbed with a force that didn't seem feasible in her withered state.

She already knew. She had known all along.

◌Over the course of the following week I noticed that something magical happened to Eileen. When I spoke to her on rounds, she heard everything I said. Her "hearing problem" had vanished. Her bizarre monotone ceased and she spoke with normal intonation and cadence. She greeted us in the mornings pleasantly and politely. She didn't whine or complain. Her childlike personality had evaporated almost entirely. Suddenly, there was a real person inside her skin.

I wouldn't ever say that a diagnosis of AIDS was a good thing for anyone, but for Eileen, it seemed a relief. She appeared so much less pained now. After months, perhaps years, she could finally come in out of the oblivion and join the ranks of the living, for whatever time she had left. She could finally afford to accept help.

None of this, of course, changed the bleak facts of an illness that was invariably terminal in the days before protease inhibitors and multi-drug therapy. She still had a horrible disease and faced a grave prognosis, but maybe her final weeks would now be a little easier. Maybe, for whatever time she had left, she could stop fighting so hard and bask in her family's obvious love.

I'm trying, Mrs. Rodriguez, I thought. I'm trying to make it better. Eileen would never live as long as Elba Rodriguez, but maybe her remaining days would be less tormented now. No matter what I could do, I couldn't prevent her death. But maybe she could take comfort in her own human dignity.

✑The calendar month ended just a few days later, and I was rotated to another ward. Eileen and her family were sad to see me leave. I was, too. But secretly, and somewhat guiltily, I was relieved. Making the diagnosis was agonizing enough—I didn't think I could handle the death.

But I continued to run into Mrs. O'Neil in the hospital hallway while rounding with my new team or waiting for the elevator. She would update me on Eileen's condition, always wanting to know my medical opinion. She still seemed to believe that I possessed special knowledge that the other doctors did not. The bags under her eyes were growing heavier, the creases on her forehead more furrowed. "The boys, you know," she would sigh. "It's not easy at my age."

I discovered that Eileen's aunt lived in the same apartment building as I did. I would see her sometimes in our lobby or doing laundry in the basement. She always offered me a smile and a polite inquiry as to my welfare before discussing Eileen.

Whenever I asked how she herself was doing, she would just smile and say "Fine, Doctor." She would never elaborate. Even after I offered her my first name—we were neighbors after all—she still insisted on addressing me as "Doctor."

Much to my surprise, Eileen made it out of the hospital, nearly six weeks after the day her priest had called the ambulance. Over that win-ter, though, she was readmitted many times. I usually ran into the aunt as she was heading out of our apartment building to go to the grocery store, with her purse strapped across her chest and her small metal shopping cart dragging behind her. I was always careful to ask something nonspecific like "How are things?" rather than "How's Eileen?" in case Eileen had died in the interim. Between these lobby conversations and what I overheard from my colleagues at work, I kept tabs on Eileen's fragile existence.

One evening that spring I was heading out of my apartment building, dressed up and excited to celebrate a friend's graduation. The party was to be in a trendy bar in SoHo, the kind that had a funky back room that you could only get into if someone knew the owner. My friend apparently did. I was practically skipping out the door when I ran straight into Mrs. O'Neil and her sister entering the portal. Their long faces and weary eyes immediately made me feel self-conscious about my festive mood and guilty about any ability to enjoy life. The aunt mentioned that she'd been in the hospital herself recently. "If I don't pay attention," she said with a wan smile, "that diabetes can really act up." I noticed that she'd lost weight and looked more haggard than I'd remembered. But before I could say anything, she touched my arm and asked how my residency training was progressing.

I was afraid to ask, but they told me, unbidden, that Eileen was back at Bellevue. She had tuberculosis and was now in an isolation room. "She doesn't really know where she is," her mother said, shaking her head. "I don't even think she recognizes us." I slunk out of the doorway, torn between my earlier exuberance and the immense sadness of these two long-suffering women. How could getting into the funky back room of a SoHo bar mean anything when somebody's beloved daughter was slipping away?

Two days later I overheard a coworker say that Eileen O'Neil had died. She had outlived my prediction by seven months, but what a painful seven months it had been. I felt it was my obligation, but also my desire, to attend her funeral.

I was sure I'd run into the aunt in my lobby to find out the details but somehow our paths did not cross that week. I tried to find out which apartment she lived in, but I realized, to my horror, that I had never learned her name. She was just Eileen's aunt. I described her to my neighbors but found that I had so few specific details in my memory other than the firm clutch with she held her purse and the smile she always managed to muster whenever she saw me. Why didn't I know more about this woman?

I didn't know Mrs. O'Neil's first name and there were too many O'Neils in the Manhattan phone book. I checked the newspaper for a funeral announcement, but there was none. By this time many days had passed and the funeral had surely taken place. After occupying such a place of respect in the family's eyes, the least I could have done was attend the funeral. That's what dedicated doctors always did on TV. But I couldn't rewind the tape—I had missed it.

After that, I was afraid to run into the family. I dreaded facing them and my shame. A few months later, however, I saw the two sisters by the mailbox in our lobby. I cringed, hoping they wouldn't notice me, but they walked toward me with smiles and warm greetings. I felt even worse. As usual, they asked about me and my family before getting to themselves. I squirmed in my shoes as they earnestly inquired about my future plans after residency.

Before they could even mention Eileen, I burst out with an apology for not attending the funeral. I felt so pathetic as I tried to explain my lame efforts to track them down. "Oh, don't worry, Doctor," they protested, smiling. "We know you have so many patients to take care of. You were so good to Eileen and we are ever grateful." I dragged myself out the door, my face burning. How could they be so generous to me?

Over the next two years I ran into the aunt periodically. We would chat about the weather and the latest rent increase. She always wanted to know how my medical training was going. One day, we found ourselves together in the laundry room. I was taking the last of my clothes from the dryer and she was starting a load of whites. Pouring in her detergent, she informed me that her sister had died four months ago.

The younger son was now in the custody of another relative. I sighed, thinking of the pain that woman must have brought to her grave. It also dawned on me that I had seen the aunt just recently in the supermarket, but she hadn't mentioned her sister's death.

Reading my mind, the aunt put down her detergent and walked over to me. She took my hand. "I know you're probably wondering why I didn't tell you the last time I saw you. I wanted to tell you, but you looked so happy that day. I remember that you were smiling and looked so pretty. I didn't want to burden you."

I didn't see the aunt very much that following year. I was busy with my life and my patients. One January evening I was hauling suitcases up to my apartment after returning from vacation. In the elevator I overheard someone saying that a woman on the sixth floor had died during the Christmas holiday. Somebody who lived alone. The maintenance man had to break down the door. Apparently, she had been dead for many days before anyone noticed.

I was suddenly gripped with panic. I ran down to the doorman. "Was she the Irish lady? Short, with gray hair, always had a smile?"

"Yeah," he sighed, "that was her. The one who was always smiling."

Three funerals; I somehow managed to miss every one.

❧Years later, when I was an attending physician at Bellevue, Mary Lou became my patient for a brief time at the Bellevue clinic when her regular doctor was on maternity leave. Mary Lou had finally retired from HIV counseling. "I'm seventy-four now," she sighed. "At my age you can't keep doing stuff like that. Too painful." She had been a regular patient at the clinic for many years, but since she was no longer working at Bellevue, she had decided to switch her medical care to a place closer to home. This was her last visit.

After I'd written her prescriptions and filled out her lab slips, we talked about Eileen. I told her what had happened to the rest of the family. And I thanked her for what she had done, both for Eileen and for me.

We shared a moment of silence for the O'Neil family. My stomach was heavy, thinking of those years of relentless suffering. I hoped that even within their pain, the mother and the aunt were able to experience a few moments of joy with their boys. I hoped that there was some sunlight in their lives.

Mary Lou gave me a big hug good-bye. I knew those arms had hugged and comforted so many people at Bellevue for so many years. I sighed and held tight for a few more minutes. It was warm and alive in there.

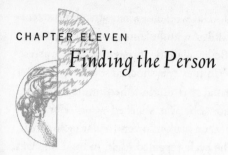

CHAPTER ELEVEN

Finding the Person

MARGARET WHITNEY was laid out in Bed 1 of the cardiac care unit when I rounded with my team on the first day of our new service. Since rounds always began in the CCU, Mrs. Whitney was the first patient we met that day. She was a pale, fleshy woman with a breathing tube jutting out of her mouth. It was fastened with white tape wrapped numerous times around her head. A feeding tube snaked out of her nose, taped to her nostrils and forehead. Multiple IV lines twisted through the bed sheets. There was a cardiac monitor on her chest, a blood pressure cuff on her arm, and a pulse-oximeter on her index finger. A urinary catheter and a rectal temperature cord exited from the sheets at the foot of her bed.

There was such a large web of white tape securing everything in place that I could barely see Mrs. Whitney—she was a mummy. What little skin peered out was an angry red, abraded from the irritation of surgical tape, with an oily glean of Vaseline that had been applied to soothe it. Her limbs were black and blue from needles and IVs. Her neck had scars from multiple central lines. Her chest was branded with two flaming rectangles, souvenirs from the paddles that had shocked her heart so many times. Her smell was a mix of antiseptic and baby powder. Her eyes drifted vacantly about the room, blinking randomly, focusing on nothing.

Mrs. Whitney, a fifty-year-old white woman from South Carolina, had been in New York City visiting her daughter. They were touring the United Nations on Mother's Day weekend when Mrs. Whitney collapsed. A bystander started CPR. An ambulance whisked her fifteen blocks down First Avenue to Bellevue in the throes of a cardiac arrest. In the emergency room Mrs. Whitney was shocked several times. Her heart briefly resumed its normal rhythm, but then immediately degenerated into electrical chaos. She was shocked again. Her heart snapped into normal rhythm, then back into ventricular tachycardia. She was shocked again and the cycle repeated itself. In total, she was shocked twenty-three times. The doctors in the ER had stopped removing the electrical paddles from her chest; they just left them lying there, simply pressing the button each time her heart went back into v-tach.

Meanwhile, her blood pressure had bottomed out. Pressors, potent intravenous medications to maintain blood pressure, were of little effect. A counter-pulsation balloon pump was threaded into her aorta to augment the pumping of her heart. Powerful anti-arrhythmic drugs were infused into every available vein.

After thirty minutes of intense work, she gradually, almost unbelievably, began to stabilize. Her heart rhythm eased into normalcy. Her heart muscle recovered from its shock and soon began to pump blood on its own. Over the next few days, the anti-arrhythmics and pressors were weaned. The aortic balloon pump was removed.

The Advanced Cardiac Life Support protocols that are droned into every intern's head had been carried out with remarkable efficiency. The paramedics, doctors, and nurses had all risen to the occasion with a heroic effort to save a young, otherwise healthy, woman. Her heart was rescued.

But for her brain, the thirty-minute resuscitation had been twenty-six minutes too long.

My team and I approached Mrs. Whitney. The intern presented a thirty-second blurb of her history that he had gotten from the previous intern last night and then we all stood in front of the bed fingering the medical tools in our pockets, eyeing the silence.

I tugged my stethoscope out from its lair. It uncurled itself as it emerged from its nest of stainless steel instruments. "Mrs. Whitney," I called out as it waggled in the air, ready and eager to extract raw data. It seemed rude not to at least address the patient before launching into the physical exam. "Good morning, Mrs. Whitney. How are you today?" My voice sounded too loud for the room. The stethoscope's wriggling petered out to a bashful stillness. I stood there stupidly, wondering how long I was supposed to wait for no answer.

I pulled back the sheet and ground my knuckles into her sternum, but she did not respond. I went through the other "arousal maneuvers"—pinching her skin, squeezing the bony brow over her eye. Mrs. Whitney's eyes continued to wander but she didn't react to any painful stimuli.

I waded through the knot of wires, tubing, and tape on her chest to find a bit of free skin upon which to place my stethoscope. It landed with a relieved plunk on her breastbone. A rhythmic bass note echoed through its tubing into my ears—her heart was beating defiantly. Her breath was steady and even, in tune with the ventilator.

I scrolled through the bedside computer—her labs had all normalized. Her chest X-rays reflected the healthy constitution of a fifty-year-old who had never smoked or been sick. Her body was strong. With a little help from the Bellevue electrical socket it had managed to recover from a massive heart attack. But Margaret Whitney wasn't there anymore.

My team stood patiently behind me, waiting for me to state the "assessment and plan" so we could move on to meet the seventeen other new patients on our service. "Well, let's...um..." I fiddled with the ventilator settings. "Let's continue current management." The buttons and dials were a relief to my hands. I twisted them around, grateful for their texture and substance. Grateful that they allowed me some action with this inanimate patient. "Let's lower her tidal volume to 500cc to avoid barotrauma. Check a blood gas in an hour and monitor her peak pressures." I hurried my team on to the next bed.

❦Mrs. Whitney, unlike many of the patients in Bellevue, wasn't homeless and had a family. Her daughter and son-in-law lived in Brooklyn. Her husband, two brothers, and one son, along with their respective spouses, had left their homes and jobs in South Carolina after the heart attack to take up residence in a nearby hotel.

I tried to keep track of everybody's names and respective relationships to Mrs. Whitney, but I kept mixing them up. They all had the same Southern accent and their conspicuously polite demeanors made it clear that they were out-of-towners. Her daughter, Sandra, was the only one I could keep straight.

Sandra was a computer consultant who had lived up north for six years and had shed much of her Southern accent and mannerisms. Her strawberry-blond hair was brushed back in an efficient, professional style, and it seemed that the brownish highlights were taking over now that she wasn't in the sun so much. She and her husband had purchased a prewar brownstone in an industrial part of Brooklyn that was rapidly gentrifying and had been restoring it for the past two years.

Renovating an old brownstone was one of my pet dreams. Whenever I saw an old, burnt-out building in the city, I would search out signs of hidden beauty—crumbled gargoyles, rusted ironwork filigree, chipped window facades. There was so much potential in every abandoned wreck. If only I had a little money and some construction know-how . . .

"Just last week we tore up two layers of linoleum in the kitchen," Sandra told me one morning as I stood by her mother's side, flushing an IV with saline. "You would not believe the beautiful hardwood floors that were hiding underneath. Long planks of oak, or maybe maple, with the original nails. It's still covered with crusted layers of glue and wax, but once we clean it . . ."

Oh, to have real hardwood floors.

"The front stoop has built-in flower boxes. Someone must have attached these flower containers to the stoop at some point, maybe in the 1940s or fifties, because they're not in the original blueprint of the house. Richard planted peonies a few weeks ago and now they're in a wild bloom."

Flowers on a front stoop. Urban flora facing off against the sea of concrete.

I took vicarious pleasure in hearing about Sandra's restoration. I was even a little jealous that someone of my generation had already purchased and renovated a house. I hadn't even left the academic womb yet.

By tradition, morning rounds always started in the CCU—sickest patients first. Mrs. Whitney was technically sick, therefore she was first, but her body was in good shape. There was actually very little for us to do.

I felt sorry for Mrs. Whitney, but from a resident point-of-view, she was a "bad hit." She wasn't going to die or get discharged in the near future, but she would require endless IVs, blood draws, EKGs, and central lines. Good practice for the interns and students, but a nightmare for me. She would never get off my service.

Each morning the team stood around with our hands jammed in our pockets. I always said good morning to Mrs. Whitney, but felt self-conscious talking into thin air. I plunked my stethoscope on her chest each day, listening with half an ear. All the information I needed was displayed on the four-color cardiac monitor. A physical exam wasn't really necessary, but I wanted to set a good example for the students.

I came to dread morning rounds because they started with Mrs. Whitney.

But afternoon rounds were different. Sandra was usually there with one or two other family members. When they were present, I made a special effort not to slack on the proprieties of bedside manner. Although for me Mrs. Whitney was merely an immobile piece of flesh buried in medical paraphernalia, I talked to her as though she could hear and understand me. I paused after each of my questions, allowing what I thought was adequate time for Mrs. Whitney to answer, if she could. I performed a more comprehensive physical exam. My team, and probably the family, was aware of the element of charade involved. It wasn't disrespectful, just a genuine effort to avoid the inevitable social carelessness around a comatose patient.

Sandra stared intently as I went through these motions. She followed my hands as they checked the pulse, then palpated the abdomen. She watched me flick the penlight in her mother's vacant eyes. She tracked the bell of my stethoscope as it traveled from Mrs. Whitney's heart, to her lungs, to her stomach. There was always tension at the end as I dislodged the stethoscope from my ears. Sandra would catch my eye, waiting for a pronouncement, as if that particular physical exam on that particular day would provide some revelation of miraculous change.

But I had nothing to say. Nothing changed. Nothing ever changed. Every day was the same. I was only going through the motions. There was no doctoring for me to do for Mrs. Whitney.

"You know," said Sandra one day, as I was adjusting the flow rate on the ventilator setting, "my mother had the best sense of humor. You should have seen her at our Christmas parties. She wouldn't have more than two sips of wine before she was rocking the house with her stories. She'd tell stories about her crazy uncle Julian and his egg farm in Shawspee. Uncle Julian and his eggs . . ." Sandra's voice trailed off and there was a long pause. "I never knew if her stories were true or not, but she charmed everyone. My father says she charmed her way into becoming the homecoming queen at their high school."

I stared at Mrs. Whitney. Her body was entangled in a web of alien tentacles. I hunted for the homecoming queen. I squinted to see the sense of humor, but there was nothing that resembled a person. I marveled at how Sandra could smile at her, touch her, talk to her as though she was there and I wished I could do the same. But she wasn't a person to me, just an object in a bed.

One afternoon I came into the CCU and Sandra grabbed me by the hand, pulling me close to the bed. "Just two minutes before you came in she looked at me when I spoke to her."

Sandra leaned over her mother and waved her hand with the eagerness of greeting a loved one at the airport. "Mom. It's me, Sandy." Mrs. Whitney's eyes meandered about the room, lofting from the IV pole to the blank ceiling corner to the red plastic needle-disposal box affixed to the wall. Sandra turned back to me. "I promise you," she said, her enthusiasm undamped, "she really looked at me when I spoke."

Sandra rubbed her mother's hand and called out to her again. "Mom, you can hear me, can't you?"

"Those eye movements are involuntary," I said quietly.

Sandra caught her breath with a panicked shiver. "With God as my witness, she looked at me." She kneaded her thumbs into her mother's palm, the flesh rippling into white and then back into pink. "She's my mother and I know when she hears me."

"I know it seems that way," I said, almost in a whisper, "but..."

"Mommy, I'm here," Sandra pleaded. "Look at me. Please ..."

I closed my eyes from the scene, unable to watch. "It's just a coincidence that her eyes sometimes move toward you when you speak. But her cortex can't process anything they're seeing. I ... I'm sorry."

∽In the ICU, whenever one of the interns would prattle on with the microscopic clinical details about an otherwise comatose or terminal patient, the resident would halt the discussion by drawing a rectangle in the air with two fingers. "The big picture," those fingers delineated. It might have looked harsh or cynical to an outsider looking in, but it was the truth. Like Dr. Schwartz who was dying of pancreatic cancer. What did it matter if his potassium was 3.3? What was being gained when we supplemented it to reach 3.7, except that the computer would no longer flag it as abnormal and the nurse would stop paging us for low potassium levels. The big picture. Not to be callous about the patient's comfort or the family's concerns. Not to relinquish the role of doctor. Not to presume any powers over life and death. Not to "play God." But the big picture.

Mrs. Whitney's brain was not going to wake up. No matter what I did, no matter what Sandra prayed for, it wasn't going to wake up. The big picture.

Every afternoon I rounded on Mrs. Whitney. But I was really rounding on Sandra. Mrs. Whitney couldn't hold up her end of the doctor-patient relationship, so her daughter slipped into that role. Our conversations were the same ones I was having with my other patients. I would ask Sandra how she was feeling today. I would review with her the results of the most recent X-rays. I would inform her of the plan for the day and comment on the weather. I'd ask about the latest update on her brownstone restoration. I felt like I was taking *her* history. At times I was tempted to listen to Sandra's lungs with my stethoscope.

It was hard for both of us to talk about the reality of what was happening. Sandra preferred to focus on the minutia of her mother's care. She wanted to know what the latest blood gas was or when we'd be doing the next pulmonary function test. My fingers quivered, aching to draw the rectangle in the air.

As the days progressed to weeks, it became increasingly evident that Mrs. Whitney would never wake up. An EEG was done to confirm her persistent vegetative state. I watched as the technician cranked up the sensitivity dial. As he wound the dial ever higher, the icy green line on the screen wavered and strained, but no recognizable waveform emerged. Though he tried different angles and alternate approaches, there was barely a blip of electrical activity in Mrs. Whitney's cortex.

Her brainstem, however, was relatively spared, which meant that the cardiovascular and respiratory centers of the brain were functioning. Her heart was able to beat independently in a normal rhythm. She could breathe on her own for several hours at a time. She would still always require a breathing tube, however, because her gag and cough reflexes were not strong enough to clear her respiratory secretions.

It was time to switch her temporary breathing and feeding tubes to permanent ones. Sandra pursed her lips and sighed when I told her this. She signed the consent forms in silence, without asking for any explanations. I wanted to ask her about her garden, but I couldn't.

In one afternoon, six different doctors worked on Mrs. Whitney in shifts. The GI team removed the feeding tube from her nose and implanted one in her abdominal wall. The ENT team removed the breathing tube from her mouth and replaced it with one that entered through a small hole in her neck.

The layers of tape on her face were finally peeled off.

Suddenly Mrs. Whitney's mouth and cheeks and forehead ap-

peared. A shock of frizzy blondish-red hair was liberated from her hel-
met of gauze and tape. A gentle-faced woman with sparkling pale blue
eyes was revealed. A new person had come to Bed 1 in place of the alien
mummy.

Sandra told me about the famous strawberry and asparagus pancakes her mother would cook up with the kids on rainy days. She told
me about the time her mother dressed up as a two-humped camel for
a PTA fund-raiser. I gazed at Mrs. Whitney's face and I could see how
an impish smile might creep in. Her eyes seemed mischievous and her
curls looked spirited. On morning rounds I didn't feel quite so self-
conscious in my one-sided conversations with Mrs. Whitney. I listened
a little harder with my stethoscope.

Once, when I was volunteering as a rape crisis counselor in my first
semester of medical school, I was called into the ER to see a young
homeless woman who had just been raped. The woman was disheveled, dirty, and powerfully malodorous. My stomach churned
when a roach sauntered out of her tattered dress. I didn't think I had
the wherewithal to overcome my disgust to do my job.

As I cringed behind the Triage desk, pretending to be involved with
paperwork, a nurse's aide approached the woman. She smoothed the
woman's matted hair. She took her dirt-encrusted hand and gently
guided her to the shower, all the while talking softly to her with a reassuring smile. I was awed and humbled.

For me, Mrs. Whitney slowly regained her humanity. I could stand
next to her and chat. I often found my hand resting on hers while I examined her lungs. I rearranged her pillows when her neck looked
kinked. She was suddenly one of my patients, one of the people that I
cared for. And I thought about Josh.

What if Josh had been "successfully" resuscitated like Mrs. Whitney.
What if he had ended up in the CCU with his twenty-seven-year-old
body whose muscles and bones were strong enough to live for decades.
I wondered if the doctors and nurses would have seen him as I'd initially seen Mrs. Whitney—as an inanimate object enmeshed in cold
wires and faceless tubes, swaddled in waves of white cloth tape. Would

they have walked by him each day with a charade of medical concern, their fingers outlining a rectangle in the air? My heart ached at the thought of my Josh being lost in the shuffle like that.

But one day, however, all the tubes would be relocated and all the tape unwound. Would one of the doctors suddenly see how warm his eyes were? Would she push the hair out of his eyes and be startled by how soft those dark curls were? Would she note the calluses on his left fingers and guess that he'd played the guitar?

I wondered if one day she would freeze in her tracks, in the middle of putting in an IV, and suddenly be hit in the stomach by the magnitude of the loss. This patient, this "bad hit," was a person. A person who'd existed in a complicated web of parents and sisters and friends, who'd had a job in midtown and an apartment with a view of the river, who had a soft spot for ice cream sundaes, who'd collected Bob Dylan albums. A person who was now gone and had left a living, gaping crater in the lives of everyone who was part of that web.

The might-have-beens and could-have-beens needled through my shoulders. I thought about the crater in Sandra's life, and in her brothers' and father's. That aching hollowness that would forever fester, even if somewhat softened over the years. A human being—a mother and a wife—had been wrenched from their lives, never to return.

℘The family meeting took place on a Thursday afternoon. Nine family members attended—probably a record at Bellevue—along with the head nurse, the social worker, the chaplain, the cardiologist, the pulmonologist, and the neurologist. We squeezed into the cramped conference room next to the CCU amidst stacks of X-rays, patient charts, medical textbooks, and aged Styrofoam coffee cups. Sandra's and Richard's hands were on the table, tightly interwoven.

Each "expert witness" presented their findings.

The focus, however, was on the neurology attending, Dr. Simmons. Her voice was direct, but gentle, with a Midwestern flavor to it. I watched as she made eye contact with each family member in turn. "Mrs. Whitney—Margaret—is in a persistent vegetative state. It's like being in a coma where you are asleep, but your heart and lungs still work. Margaret is a strong woman and she could possibly live this way for a very long time."

Dr. Simmons tucked a few errant strands of her short red hair behind her ear. "I know everyone has heard stories about people waking up after ten years. Unfortunately that's not the way it really happens. Once the cortex of the brain—the thinking part—is damaged from lack of oxygen, it isn't able to recover. That part of the brain is dead."

I thought about the stories that Sandra had told me about the strawberry and asparagus pancakes, and the two-humped camel. From my spot in the corner, I watched Richard place his left hand over Sandra's, which was already cradled in his right. Their matching wedding rings shimmered from the reflected fluorescent lights.

Everyone's eyes were fixed on Dr. Simmons. I noticed that in addition to red hair, she also had freckles, just like Mrs. Whitney. "At this point," Dr. Simmons said softly, but firmly, "I don't think she needs to be in the hospital. I think she would be better served in a nursing facility." She invited the family to ask questions and answered every one, even the ones that were repetitive, without ever seeming impatient. In my head, I whispered a "thank you" to Dr. Simmons for doing this difficult job that I'd so dreaded.

Finally, the room grew silent. The family members looked at each other grimly and the expert witnesses stared down at their laps. I realized that people were waiting for the meeting to end and were looking to me to do it. I fingered my stethoscope nervously. "I guess we can all see the situation now," I stammered. "It doesn't appear that Mrs. Whitney is going to wake up. I think we have done all we can for her." I winced at what sounded like stock dialogue from a cheap movie. Sandra had started weeping softly in the back and Richard was rubbing her shoulder. "I know this has been so hard on all of you," I said. "I wish we had something better to say. I wish . . ." Sandra was sobbing out loud now. I missed Josh desperately.

✑The next day we began the arduous task of transferring Mrs. Whitney to a nursing home in South Carolina. The logistics were a nightmare (how *do* you transfer a patient on a breathing machine from New

York to South Carolina, and who pays for it?). In a city hospital with limited social services, it fell to the residents to do most of the social work. I filled out stacks of forms and spent hours on the phone with various agencies. After four weeks of faxing and telephoning and wading through interminable bureaucracy, Mrs. Whitney finally went home to South Carolina.

I said good-bye to Sandra and her mother in the CCU. By plan or by coincidence, the CCU and ICU have enormous picture windows that look out over the East River. The unconscious patients of Bellevue have views of the water that real estate tycoons would kill for. Josh's apartment had the same view. The bright June sun sparkled over the river into the CCU, casting silver reflections off the stainless steel ventilators. Sandra and I gazed out of the window for a few minutes without speaking. I didn't have any words of inspiration or wisdom to pass on, and I guess she didn't expect any. We smiled half-smiles and shook hands slowly.

∽Mrs. Whitney is probably still alive today, given her basically healthy fifty-year-old body. I hope that the staff members at her nursing home are as courageously compassionate as that nurse's aide I'd watched in the ER with the homeless woman. I hope they are as loving as Sandra and her family would be. I hope they treat her as I would have wanted Josh to be treated. I hope they wash her gently, smooth her hair, and talk softly to her while they change her sheets. I hope they remain respectful that perhaps somewhere, locked inside Mrs. Whitney's body, are remnants of a life—of learning to ride a bicycle, of giving birth to a child, of the smell of a South Carolina meadow. I hope they act with the sense that Mrs. Whitney could be their mother, or daughter, or sister. I hope they find the person within the patient.

CHAPTER TWELVE

Positive

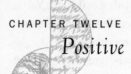

I mean, however and wherever we are,
We must live as if we will never die.

Nazim Hikmet, "On Living"

SHE WAS A TINY WOMAN, but she had me cornered near the 16-West nurses' station, practically grabbing the lapels of my white coat. "Are you accusing my niece of having AIDS?" she hissed, her face only inches from mine. "My niece doesn't do drugs, she doesn't hang around nasty people, she's never had any bad diseases. She's a good girl!"

Her voice began to rise as she pressed closer into me and the sing-song of her Jamaican accent became more dissonant. "You doctors think every Black or Hispanic kid who comes in here has AIDS. I've been at Bellevue for twenty-five years and I've seen how you doctors are." The gray strands in her black hair shimmered with rage. "Don't you ever talk to my niece like that again." By now she was nearly screaming. "And you're only a resident! I want her transferred to a real doctor."

I tried to edge backward, but she locked her glare on me and I couldn't move. Her angry breath seared the skin on my face. "I don't trust you," she said, plunging one firm finger into my chest. "Stay away from my niece!"

A few people stuck their heads out of offices to see what all the commotion was. I mustered my most diplomatic voice. "Mrs. Stanton, I'm not saying that Yvette definitely has HIV. It's just that the type of pneumonia she has can be associated with HIV."

"Don't give me no a-sso-ci-a-tions." She sputtered each syllable at me. "I know my niece and she does not have AIDS."

I lowered my voice. "I'm not trying to say anything bad about Yvette. It's just that in the chance she does have HIV, we should know now so she can get the most effective and appropriate treatments."

"The 'appropriate treatment' is for you to stop harassing her about taking that AIDS test. My niece does not have AIDS. Period." She paused and shifted her posture so that her head was cocked even closer to me. I could see right down the part in the middle of her head. "Do you hear me? Period!"

∽It was only last week that I had been scrutinizing Yvette's chest X-ray in the cramped radiology room in the ER. All the normal lung markings were scrunched up like a crumpled newspaper. It was as though she hadn't taken a deep enough breath to expand the alveoli of her lungs. True, Yvette was short of breath, but she didn't strike me as sick enough to explain these dense markings on the X-ray. I marched over to her stretcher. "This X-ray isn't good enough," I announced. "We're doing it again, but this time take a real breath!"

The second X-ray was essentially unchanged. The crowded lung markings could have been ordinary pneumonia or might have been consistent with PCP (pneumocystis) pneumonia. Yvette just didn't seem like AIDS to me. Something didn't fit.

I waded back through the noise and general chaos of the ER to take Yvette's history. With her silky complexion, large luminous eyes, and generous supply of baby fat, she barely looked sixteen. But she was panting. I could see her gulping for air between sentences and a slender line of moisture framed her forehead. The muscles of her neck and chest walls weren't straining, though, so I wasn't worried she was going to "crap out" and need a breathing tube.

"It's only recently, doctor. Maybe a few weeks ago that I started feeling like I have asthma. I've never been sick ... ever." Yvette paused, adjusting the oxygen tubing that opened into her nose. She inhaled heavily. "With the cold weather, and all.... it's making me feel like an old person."

I asked her if she'd been a physically active person before these symptoms started. "Well, not exactly," Yvette said with a chuckle. "As you can see, I have a few pounds to lose. But I," she stopped for a breath, "I get around fine. My two little ones keep me moving.

"This breathing stuff just knocked me out. I mean, in the last few days, what with Christmas and New Year's. All the guests and everything . . . I could barely make it across the kitchen floor." Her voice rose for emphasis, but then she had to pause for a breath. "My aunt—we live with my aunt—kept telling me to come to Bellevue, but I've never needed any doctors. I've always been healthy. You probably know my aunt . . . she works over in Medical Records. She knows *everybody* at Bellevue." Yvette rolled her eyes and managed a sarcastic grin.

Yvette told me that she was interested in becoming a paralegal. She had graduated high school and was contemplating college, but was now raising her children full time. She blushed when I questioned her about risk factors for HIV. She had never used drugs, never received any blood transfusions, and did not have multiple sexual partners.

When I asked about the man who was the father of her children, her tone hardened and dropped in pitch. "Him? He's long gone from my life. I don't want to know from nothing about him."

I paused, debating if I should pursue this. "Can you tell me just a little about him," I ventured. "Was he generally healthy?"

Yvette shrugged and her gaze strayed over to the green oxygen tank standing near her stretcher.

"Do you know if he ever did drugs or had a blood transfusion?"

"Listen, I have nothing to do with him," she said flatly, her eyes fixed on the oblong tank. "He's not part of my life."

"I know these questions are uncomfortable, but they are important."

Yvette continued staring at the oxygen tank with the pressure monitors and warning signs attached to it.

"Do you know if he had a lot of other partners?" I asked.

"He is out of my life. He doesn't exist." She pulled her eyes back and they landed hard and heavy on me. "Can we just get back to me already?"

I nodded—I'd gone too far. "You're right. I'm sorry. We'll stay with you."

I looked at the X-ray again with its bunched-up lung markings. Could this be PCP or was it just garden-variety pneumonia that could be easily treated with erythromycin? In my gut I did not think that Yvette had AIDS. Her history wasn't consistent with HIV and she didn't have "the look," like Eileen O'Neil had. She was, if anything, overweight. Her skin glowed with youthful health. This didn't smell of AIDS. To reinforce my feelings, and perhaps to convince those around me, I ordered the first dose of erythromycin to be given stat.

But just to be sure, I wanted to repeat the X-ray one more time.

I hauled Yvette back to radiology. Ignoring the technician's complaints about three chest X-rays in one hour, I hounded Yvette like a football coach. "Okay," I said, "this is it! This time you are going to take a deeper breath. The deepest breath in the world. Stretch out those lungs! Get that air in! Breathe!"

I was back in the tiny radiology room again, squished between the dented metal desk and the lumbering file cabinets, staring at the third X-ray. Two other residents were jostling me for the same lightbox to read their films. I tried to will Yvette's lung markings apart. I ordered them to disengage, to separate, to untwist, to disconnect. But they wouldn't budge. I flipped the X-ray back and forth. I scrutinized it under the extra bright "hot light." I blocked the heart image with my palm to eliminate distracting shadows. I varied the ambient lighting. I squinted and covered my weaker eye. I removed my glasses and pressed the X-ray right up to my nose. But it was no use. The lung markings wouldn't part.

Harrison's Principles of Internal Medicine lists forty diseases that can present with "increased interstitial lung markings," but in New York City in the early 1990s there was only one. I couldn't deny it any longer.

I slunk back to the ER and with painful, reluctant penmanship, switched Yvette's antibiotic from erythromycin to Bactrim, the most effective drug for PCP. I lowered my eyes as I wrote the order, avoiding the "I told you so" stare from the ER nurse.

"I can't be sure exactly which type of pneumonia you have," I explained to Yvette, "until we do a bronchoscopy to get a lung biopsy. But I am concerned that you might have PCP. PCP pneumonia occurs in illnesses that suppress the immune system."

"What kind of illnesses do that?" Yvette asked, looking straight at me.

"Well," I said, trying to sound nonchalant, "if you are on chemotherapy or steroids. Cancer could do it." I swallowed. "And HIV could do it, too."

Yvette continued to stare directly at me, but didn't say anything.

I lowered my voice to a whisper. "I think you should do an HIV test." Yvette pursed her lips and shook her head firmly.

⋙Yvette had improved surprisingly fast after she was started on Bactrim. She continued to refuse the bronchoscopy and the HIV test, but within a few days she was breathing normally and was able to walk around without oxygen.

Aside from our daily disagreement on morning rounds over testing, we got along well. I never got to meet Yvette's kids because they were too young to come up to the wards, but she told me how Stephan babbled nonstop on the phone. Apparently his great-aunt was reading extra stories to him at night so he really didn't miss his mother all that much. Sarah was just learning how to talk and was a little intimidated by the phone, but she was having fun with the snow.

Yvette had an easy affability about her and a catchy smile. When she grinned, two capacious dimples illuminated her face and you couldn't help but smile back. The three older women who shared her room became stand-in grandmothers, boasting about Yvette's progress to all the other patients on the ward. Yvette's nightstand was piled high with the cookies and candies they hoarded for her.

⋙While an HIV test required consent, a T-cell test did not (at least at that time). T-cells are the white blood cells most affected by HIV. Normally, humans possess well over a thousand T-cells in a milliliter of blood. Less than 500 is typically when HIV treatment is begun, even though patients are usually asymptomatic. Below 200 is when most opportunistic infections begin. Without Yvette's consent, we sent her blood sample for a T-cell count. On the day after her discharge it came back at 8.

That evening I bundled up and walked down to Little India on East Sixth Street. The block was lined with all manner of Indian and Pakistani restaurants, crammed one against the next. Sitar music and curry fragrances wafted along the entire stretch. Brash lights in raucous multicolor festooned the windows all year round, but at this time of year tourists could be forgiven for assuming that these were in honor of Christmas.

The restaurants were virtually interchangeable. They proffered identical menus, the same assortments of *biryani, tandoori,* and *vindaloo* printed in the same script in the same order. *Saag panir* and fluffy *poori* bread were indistinguishable from one to the next. The only one that stood out for me was the one that was on the south side of the street closest to Second Avenue—the one that had been Josh's favorite. Josh was convinced that Passage to India served better food than the others, but we all knew that it was because his buddy always gave Josh (and his friends) a free mixed appetizer plate. That restaurant I couldn't bear to go into.

I stomped the snow off my boots and popped into one of the others with the intention of sitting down for a meal. But my mind felt restless and resisted the confinement. I ordered a samosa to go and continued down the block. How was I going to tell Yvette? What actual words could I use?

I could keep hinting until she figured it out. *Yvette, remember what I said about that certain kind of pneumonia? The kind that can happen when the immune system isn't working so well?* That was too horribly vague and ambiguous. I would hate for a doctor to talk to me like that. She deserved the respect of clarity, didn't she?

I swung around the corner to Eighth Street, otherwise known as St. Mark's Place. Brightly lit souvenir emporiums jutted onto the sidewalks hawking T-shirts, leather vests, silver chains, and fake Rolexes. The café on the corner offered tattoo-and-cappuccino specials.

I could be blunt and lay it on the table. *Yvette, you have AIDS.* That would certainly eliminate any ambiguity. I started on my samosa, which had grown cold by this time. *You have AIDS.* There was a leaden thud to those words. In theory it seemed easy; just speak the truth. But the truth was so awful. It was a declaration of war on Yvette's life. How could I look into those liquidy brown eyes and say that? How could I possibly launch those bellicose words? The outer layer of the samosa, now that it was no longer hot, had turned to greasy mush. The potato filling was bland without the heat to energize it. A knish by any other name was just a knish.

I stopped in front of one of the jewelry displays. Delicate diamond studs sat side by side with burly metal chains sporting pendants of skulls and daggers. Should I ease her in slowly? Should I be direct? Should I couch it in clinical terminology? Should I have a psychiatrist in the room with me? Should I ask my attending to do it?

I picked up a pair of earrings with small circles of pewter. It reminded me of the jewelry I used to buy in the Arab markets of Jerusalem, with the pressed copper discs that the vendors swore were actual ancient coins. I still had a few in my possession that I had purchased—bargained for—when I was fourteen. I held the pair in my hands, tracing the fine floral patterns that were etched into the metal. They glinted in the yellowish light of the street lamp. I closed my palm around the earrings, feeling the chill of the metal eat into my flesh.

No matter which method I chose there would be that one sentinel moment when the true meaning of my words would become evident. It almost wouldn't matter what my approach had been. Once it became apparent that I was telling Yvette that she had AIDS, all of my carefully selected words would tumble to the wayside. No matter what poets might say about the power of words, the most delicate and thoughtful prose is quashed by the leaden weight of a terminal illness.

I slipped the earrings back onto the table. My stomach was lurching from the grease of the samosa and my ears were beginning to sting from the cold. I plodded back up Second Avenue, my feet scratching against the salt that had been sprinkled on the sidewalks.

✑The night before Yvette's appointment with me in the outpatient clinic, I stayed up late memorizing different versions of my speech. I was determined to be straightforward with her. It was the least I could do, I thought. In the tempest of unknowns and fears that I imagined would ensnare anyone given a diagnosis of AIDS, I wanted to be a ballast of comfort. I wanted to have the *equinimatas* that Osler spoke of, to provide emotional support to my patient by being clear and steady. I sat with a pencil, scribbling on the back of an envelope. I erased and rewrote my lines, then erased again. I telephoned all of my friends who were psychologists and social workers. Everybody had a different opinion, but they were unanimous in their relief that *they* didn't have to do it. I jotted a new speech down. I would be honest and forthright, but not harsh. I snatched my *Roget's Thesaurus* from the shelf, tearing through the pages to find the right words; they had to exist in there somewhere. "You will find words and phrases to express all the shades and modifications of that idea," the back jacket of my 1975 edition promised. Compassion, honesty, reliability—I looked them all up. Ambiguity—I checked the antonyms. I dug through the elaborately delineated categories that Peter Mark Roget, himself a physician, had teased out of the English language a hundred years ago.

When I arrived at clinic the next day Yvette and her aunt were already waiting for me. My eyes felt too heavy to keep open and I'd been too nauseous to eat anything for breakfast. "Well . . . you see," I started, trying to control the sour gurgitations in my stomach. Suddenly I couldn't remember any of the carefully planned speech that I had memorized. "Certain types of pneumonia . . . well different types of pneumonia . . . occur with different types of immune systems." My tongue seemed disengaged from my speech; its movements consistently one step out of sync with my words. "If T-cells . . . one of the important parts of the immune system . . . aren't, you know, working so well, or aren't around in enough numbers . . ." I could feel myself drift-ing into babble. What happened to clarity and unambiguity?

Yvette began to weep softly as my tongue garbled convoluted clauses about lymphocyte ratios and seroconversion. Mrs. Stanton's breathing started to grow heavy, then became raspy and asthmatic as I felt my-self choking over antibody reactions and Western blots. Mrs. Stanton heaved into loud sobs and my throat ground down, twisting to a halt around lymphadenopathy and interstitial pneumonia. I stood there frozen, my fists plunged deep inside the pockets of my white coat. My eyes twitched around the small room, from the blood pressure cuff to the exam table to the stack of yellow X-ray request forms. Nothing would move; nothing would step forward to rescue me. I tried again to speak, but nothing would emerge—just a hoarse stutter that wilted against my teeth.

Tears began their ascent. Inside the pocket my left hand clutched the bell of the stethoscope. I coddled it between my fingers, absorbing the cool smoothness of the stainless steel. They climbed steadily, the tears, steadfastly ignoring my plea to stay down. The clammy pulse of my palm evaporated the metal coolness of the stethoscope. The tears con-tinued to push forward and the metal bell grew sticky from my heat. The tears bulged past the knot of muscles in my throat, overrunning the vise of gritted teeth. They rose in a pitch, rumbling forward, bar-reling upward, insistent in their path, until they hit their peak and spilled over.

And then there was the strange harmony of three people crying, each caught in a private dissonance. The room strained and the walls grew heavy around my head. But there was a relief in the absence of words. A relief to escape tongue-twisting jargon, those lumbering, multisyllabic words intoned from textbooks, thesauruses, and profes-sors; polyphonous clinical terms that were supposed to capture the essence of the disease. Words that I'd rehearsed and memorized, words that I'd thought would clarify and explain, but in fact served only to stymie. It was a relief to escape their tyranny and to lapse, for a moment, into the sanctuary of the nonverbal world—a world that required only the physical lexicon of the body. We cried together, sharing a language that paid no heed to linguistic proprieties, socioeconomic differences, or ethnic barriers.

Then I gingerly brought up the subject of her children and the need to get them tested. "No," said Yvette, her tears drying up. "I will not interrupt their lives. I will not allow them to be tested." When I mentioned that we should also contact her ex-boyfriend, she became furious. "I probably got it from him. I hope he dies a slow and painful death!"

ॐYvette came regularly to all of her clinic appointments. She was by far my most reliable patient. She was scrupulous about her complex regimen of medications. She called me for refills well before her current prescriptions ran out. She remembered to do her blood tests every six weeks to the day, even when I forgot. And she always had a warm, dimpled smile for me, sometimes accompanied by homemade brownies or a bag of red seedless grapes that she knew were my favorite.

We never did do the HIV test. In fact we never even used the words HIV or AIDS. Yvette couldn't bring herself to say them, and nor, I found, could I. At the beginning of each visit when I'd ask her how she was doing she would reply, "I feel fine. If you didn't tell me that I was sick, I wouldn't know that I was sick." And with the pearly glow in her cheeks and her perfect-teeth smile, it was hard to argue.

She continued to refuse an HIV test for her children. I asked her to please let me at least speak with her pediatrician, but she said no.

Just like with Dr. Schwartz, I felt pulled in different directions and wasn't sure to whom my responsibilities were. There was no chapter on this in *Harrison's* either. I conferred with several attendings about this issue and opinion was mixed. I finally consulted our legal affairs advisor. Regarding her children, it seemed, disclosure was not only possible but could even be required.

I confronted Yvette at our next visit. "I know this is a difficult thing to have to think about, especially now when there is so much on your mind, but there are a lot of people who potentially can be affected by this."

Yvette looked over to the "Children of Bellevue" poster on the wall.

"Listen, I can't force your children to be tested, but I do have the legal authority to call the pediatrician and tell him or her about your health status."

Yvette continued to stare at the poster. It was a calendar from three years ago with brightly colored children's drawings decorating the twelve months of the year.

"I'm prepared to do that," I paused for a breath, "but I'd much prefer if I had your permission." I felt like I was cornering Yvette, and I didn't like having to do that.

I saw Yvette's eyes wander from January down to June, past the blue and green snowmen over to the vibrant orange flowers. Then down to her lap. "Okay," she mumbled, barely audibly. "You win."

∽Once I'd taken care of the initial needs for Yvette—getting all of her medicines in order, setting up a regular schedule for blood tests, filling out all the Medicaid forms, talking to the pediatrician—there was suddenly a lull. We didn't have a whole lot to talk about during our visits. Especially since she felt perfectly fine. I had more time to ponder, and a fear began to grow in me. Yvette seemed so healthy now, but she could get sicker and possibly die during the course of my residency.

In some ways Yvette was so similar to Eileen—young, single mother of two, HIV acquired without drugs or needles, yet they couldn't be more different. Eileen had already been so visibly sick when I'd first met her. With her gaunt face and sallow skin, she'd already had her "terminal illness" label pinned upon her. Her arms were black and blue, and she had long since given up complaining about the needle sticks. Eileen lived in her hospital bed, permanently attired, in my mind, in a saggy blue gown and regulation green Styrofoam slippers. She was a perpetual patient for me—*only* a patient—and nothing else. I had never seen her as a healthy, functioning person and, frankly, I couldn't even envision her out in the world wearing real clothes, riding the subway, paying taxes.

Most of my clinic patients, on the other hand, were relatively healthy. They had hypertension, arthritis, or back pain. During our clinic appointments they'd tell me about a daughter graduating high school, or how long the wait at the pharmacy was, or what a lousy job the mayor was doing. We never had to discuss chemotherapy or DNRs. Maybe I'd fiddle with their blood pressure pills or remind them to get a mammogram, but I never had to think about CPR or breathing machines. The vast majority would amble along without any major medical catastrophes. And when I finished residency, I would pass them along to a new intern in basically the same condition that I'd inherited them.

But Yvette straddled both worlds. Now that she had fully recovered from her PCP, she seemed as healthy as my other clinic patients, if not more so because of her youth. But there was a high probability of her getting cryptococcal meningitis or tuberculosis or lymphoma or AIDS dementia or any of the other brutal illnesses that follow HIV's coattails. My residency might trace an unending series of medical disasters for Yvette, each one wrenching her condition down another notch. Each one sapping her hold on life. Each one driving home the point that in those days everyone with AIDS died in the near future no matter how young or how healthy they started out. During the course of my tenure at Bellevue I might have to watch Yvette wither away from this robust woman sitting in my office to one of those skeletons that limped around on the AIDS ward upstairs on 17-West.

I cringed recalling my rotation on 17-West. There was a set of dice in the doctors' station that had been fashioned out of surgical tape by some resident and pressed into cubical shapes. One die had diagnoses scribbled on each face: PCP, cryptococcal meningitis, toxoplasmosis, tuberculosis, syphilis, and Kaposi's sarcoma. The other die had prognoses: failure to thrive, DNR, coma, intubation, ICU, and the euphemistically titled ECU ("extended" care unit). For each new admission, the on-call team would roll the dice to see which combination of diagnosis and prognosis would be predicted. Points were accumulated if the dice accurately foretold the outcome.

ᴄᴏBut the months progressed and I continued to see Yvette in my clinic. We reviewed her medications, refilled prescriptions, but there wasn't a lot to do because she felt so well and her blood counts were relatively stable. Several times I offered to transfer her to the HIV clinic where she could benefit from seeing the AIDS experts. She could also enroll in clinical trials for the newest experimental medications. But Yvette would have nothing of it. She wanted to stay right here in the regular medicine clinic, with the healthy people.

I wasn't going to escape.

Occasionally, I ran into Mrs. Stanton in the hallway or down in the medical records department. We now had a strong working relationship, united in a common goal. She often brought me forms from Yvette that required my signature, and I frequently gave her prescriptions to save Yvette a trip to the clinic.

Yvette didn't acquire any other opportunistic infections. She never even caught a cold. I felt rather ridiculous writing "23-year-old Black female with HIV, T-cells = 8" at the top of each of my clinic notes, when this woman with sparkling eyes and dimples in her baby-soft cheeks was sitting in front of me. She didn't look anything like the emaciated AIDS patients on 17-West. In fact, she was concerned about being overweight and wanted to know if I could prescribe her diet pills.

Maybe Yvette was the exception to the rule. Maybe her HIV wouldn't kill her. Maybe she didn't actually have AIDS. After all, we never *did* do the HIV test. I savored that thought in my head for several weeks. I even went so far as to ask one of the immunology professors if maybe a person with eight T-cells and PCP pneumonia could have something other than AIDS. She rolled her eyes at me and I hung my head.

✑Miraculously, Yvette never felt weak or sick during the three years of my residency. Her cheeks never lost their rosy luster. Our frequent clinic visits seemed almost absurd for someone who looked so well. We religiously reviewed her blood test results, prescribed new medications as they became available, kept track of her Medicaid benefits, and updated her files as necessary. Yet we never uttered the words HIV or AIDS. I found myself guiltily joining her in euphemistic gymnastics. I sometimes even "forgot" to do a physical exam during her clinic visits.

Yvette wasn't going to die.

The end of my residency was drawing near and I gingerly brought up the issue of setting Yvette up with a new doctor. I once again offered her a referral to the HIV clinic, but she wouldn't hear of it. She preferred to stay in the regular medicine clinic. She did, after my endless badgering, agree to enroll in the NYU/Bellevue AIDS clinical trials. I was happy because it would keep her in contact with the HIV experts, even if they weren't her primary doctors.

After one of our visits I went out to the waiting room to give her some prescriptions that she had forgotten. She was there with Sarah and Stephan, now three and five. They were healthy, bouncy children, and they did not have HIV.

Yvette introduced them to me and they seemed to intuit that I was someone important in their mother's life. Sarah climbed into my lap and Stephan leaned in close to me. We spent fifteen minutes talking and drawing pictures while Yvette filled her prescriptions. Sarah introduced me to Dino, her teddy bear, and told me in a confident voice that he did not like broccoli one bit. Stephan drew a picture of a woman with a black bag and said, "That's Dr. Ofri with her doctor bag." I felt honored to be accepted into their little world so readily, as though I had always been a member. I held them in my arms, breathing in their sweetness, but overcome with guilt. They could not know that the seminal event of their grade-school years would be watching their mother grow sicker and sicker and eventually die.

I felt partially responsible for their incipient loss of a mother. I had somehow initiated the process, but I wasn't going to be there for the end; Yvette's strong constitution had spared me the worst. I was going to abandon ship before things got messy. Part of me was secretly glad that I wasn't going to witness the ugly death that HIV brings. If my final memory of Yvette was as a robust, healthy woman, I could maintain my end of the denial game.

I suddenly thought about Dr. Schwartz. About how he was so insistent in his denial. Maybe he needed that to survive. Maybe I needed *my* denial to survive—I couldn't bear to watch Yvette shrivel and die. I'd always scorned the conventional wisdom that doctors shouldn't get emotionally involved with their patients. That view seemed so archaic and paternalistic. But wasn't I doing something even worse—taking care of my patient when things were easy, but then skipping out when the hard stuff came?

There was a gravelly sensation in my stomach, opaque and acid. The logic that my departure was strictly due to the termination of residency lurched about with my guilty relief about leaving before things got messy. I was deserting Yvette—if not physically or practically, then psychologically. Was this the type of doctor I wanted to become?

And I was mortified that any relief about escaping before the hard part could possibly slither into my head as I sat with Yvette's precious children in my arms, but it did. How could I be permitted to inhale their delicate talcum fragrances or stroke their milky-soft skin when I knew I was abandoning ship? A fantasy flickered that I could adopt Stephan and Sarah after Yvette died, but they had their great-aunt, who would raise them with a fierce devotion I could never possess.

∽I dreaded my last appointment with Yvette. For the whole month I had been saying emotional good-byes to my clinic patients and I was already drained. I felt that I was abandoning them all. Yvette and I spent much of our final visit reviewing paperwork for the transition. I didn't bother with a physical exam. We studiously avoided eye contact until the very end.

"Please call me," Yvette said, "if you ever come back to Bellevue."

I was touched. We gave each other a big, satisfying bear hug before she left. Tears were in both of our eyes as we retreated to our respective sides of the clinic door. I took a few deep breaths and splashed some cold water on my face. The next patient was already in the room waiting to see me.

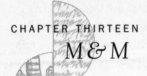

CHAPTER THIRTEEN

M & M

But from these bitter truths I must return
To my own history.

William Wordsworth, *The Prelude*, Book Eleventh

THE BODY WASN'T EVEN COLD when they informed me that I would be presenting the case at M & M. For the next forty-eight hours I clawed at the minutia of the chart, trying to absorb every laboratory value and X-ray report. I was already hallucinating blood gas numbers and ventilator settings. My intestines were roiling from caffeine.

I had never killed anyone before, so I didn't know what to expect. I mean, I had been to M & M before, but never as victim. One year, in a brief fit of morbid quaintness, the chiefs actually passed around M&M's candies at morbidity and mortality rounds.

Lord.

I hesitated at the door, determined to control my hyperventilation. The heat was building up under my stiff white coat and I could feel my skin growing sticky. I made a damp grab at the doorknob.

The conference room was already packed, but it wasn't the usual crowd of scruffy medical students and overtired residents. It was all attendings—all real doctors. I scanned the assemblage of gastroenterologists, cardiologists, radiologists, surgeons, and critical care attendings. I saw junior attendings, senior attendings, division heads, nursing supervisors, and hospital administrators. There was even someone from legal affairs. There were so many levels of hierarchy in the room that I couldn't keep track of who feared whom the most.

The case summary was gripped in my right hand, a cup of coffee in my left. Only a few drops spilled onto the typed sheets as I squirmed into my seat under the weight of their stares.

I wasn't the only person who had made the error, but as medical consult—the senior medical resident—I'd been in charge. Well, since this was University Hospital, the attending was really in charge, so I guess he'd be at the top of the lawsuit. And there were all those consultants on the case, too. But it's always the resident who gets flayed for the screwups. Residents are cheap labor for the private attendings. We carry out their orders, do all their scut, but have little say in the important medical decisions like we do at Bellevue. Of course when something goes wrong, who gets tossed into the fire at M & M? After all, this is an academic institution and we're all here to learn!

Killing a patient. Just a couple of months before the end of residency. What a way to launch a career in medicine. I had hoped for some salvation this morning, maybe a collision with the First Avenue bus on my way to the hospital, but no such reprieve was forthcoming.

The head of the department uttered some platitudes about how this session was intended to be a learning experience. I felt faint. He nodded at me to begin.

A sour taste came up in my throat, but no voice. I stared straight at the page, coaxing my vocal cords. The buzz of the fluorescent lights swarmed in my head. I quickly sipped my coffee, realizing too late that I'd forgotten to add sugar. The bitterness smarted on my tongue and finally some dry words emerged.

✐ "Mr. H is a thirty-one-year-old white male who attempted suicide three years prior to admission by ingesting a bottle of lye. His esophagus was destroyed, but a piece of colon was surgically inserted between his mouth and stomach. Periodically he experienced esophageal strictures, but they were easily opened with balloon dilatation and he had no difficulty eating or drinking. He had no other medical history and his only medication was an antidepressant.

"Last Wednesday he was admitted to University Hospital with symptoms of nausea, vomiting, and dizziness. His admission labs were within normal limits. On Thursday, endoscopy showed esophageal strictures. On Friday he underwent successful balloon dilatation of the strictures. By Saturday the patient was already able to swallow soft foods."

I was medical consult at UH that weekend. As the senior medical resident I was responsible for all the interns and residents on call. I had to handle all admissions and transfers, and of course any codes. I was irritable just having to be there—I preferred to work at Bellevue. Maybe Bellevue didn't have as many amenities, but at least we residents got to make all the decisions about patient care. At UH we had to ask the attendings permission for every little thing. It was bad enough when I was an intern taking care of Dr. Schwartz and didn't know that much medicine, but as medical consult, when I finally knew what I was doing, it was annoying and insulting.

"Later that morning the covering GI attending (Mr. H's regular doctor was off for the weekend) was called at home because the patient was hypotensive. Systolic blood pressure was in the 80s, whereas the patient's baseline pressure had been 100 to 110. The attending gave a phone order from home to administer intravenous fluids."

Weekends at UH were the worst. Thirty hours of roaming this infernal place. Everybody was old and sick and in a bad mood. The nurses were crabby on weekends. The attendings hated to be disturbed at home. I had an old bunk bed to sleep on, with sagging springs and sheets that usually smelled like the previous resident. Luckily, I suppose, I rarely had time to use it.

"Later that afternoon the intern was called to see the patient because the blood pressure was still low despite IV fluids. At that time the patient complained only of mild nausea and some dizziness when standing. The intern documented a blood pressure of 81/59 and a slightly elevated pulse of 110. There was no fever and the patient was breathing comfortably. On physical exam the patient was noted to have minimal abdominal tenderness. Labs were drawn, including a blood gas. Portable X-rays were ordered."

The intern caught up with me at the elevator at six P.M. on Saturday. "I don't know about this guy," he said to me. "His pressure's still low, but he looks great and says he feels fine. I don't know what to make of it. Could you swing by and check it out?" I gulped down my coffee and we went together to see the patient.

The smell of sickness wasn't so strong in Mr. Herlan's room—he hadn't been there long enough. The New York Times was spread out on the bed and I could see that he'd already finished the crossword puzzle. Saturday's puzzle! I was impressed. A half-empty bottle of ginger ale sat on the nightstand. My left hand probed Mr. Herlan's belly as we spoke. He was a slender white man with dark hair, dark eyes, and finely chiseled features.

"Really, Doc," he said, "I feel okay. I'm a little dizzy, a little nauseous, but it's no different than I've felt all week."

"The X-rays were within normal limits. The white count, electrolytes, and hematocrit were unchanged from baseline. But the lactate was elevated at 6.8."

Damn, 6.8! Elevated lactate meant that something was brewing somewhere. Somewhere in his body there were tissues that weren't getting enough oxygen and the cells were forced to start producing lactate. Mr. Herlan certainly didn't look as sick as his lactate suggested, but I had learned the hard way never to trifle with elevated lactates. Something bad was going on.

What could be causing the elevated lacate in Mr. Herlan? Maybe the balloon procedure from yesterday had ruptured his esophagus. Or maybe it had caused a few "micro-perforations," enough to allow intestinal bacteria to seep into his bloodstream and spread an infection. Or maybe something totally unrelated to the balloon procedure was going on. Any one of a hundred bad things could raise the lactate. But once the lactate was elevated, things could turn sour quickly. Based on his blood tests, X-rays, and physical exam, I couldn't really say what exactly was percolating under his skin, but I sure as hell wasn't going to stand around doing nothing with a lactate of 6.8.

I called the covering GI attending at home to ask if I could move Mr. Herlan to the intensive care unit. No attending at UH ever wants to get sued—he said okay.

"The patient was started on triple antibiotics to cover for possible infection. He was transferred to the ICU at seven P.M. with a blood pressure of 77/54. The patient was anxious, but he was mentally alert and had good urine output. He had no other specific complaints except mild nausea. His temperature remained normal."

Mr. Herlan pestered me as we wheeled his stretcher down the hall. "Why do I have to go to the ICU? It's only a little upset stomach. I've had this a million times before. Ginger ale and Mylanta usually do the trick. Maybe we should just wait a little longer and see if it gets better." He twisted his head on the pillow so that he could see me better. "I'm not really that sick, am I?"

Why do patients always ask these questions? How can you answer honestly without scaring them? Nobody goes to the ICU because they're healthy! But at least he's talking and urinating. If his blood pressure—low as it is—is sufficient to send oxygen to his brain and kidneys, then things can't be too bad.

I leaned over to Mr. Herlan as we waited for the service elevator. "I'm concerned about your low blood pressure. The fact that you feel okay is an excellent sign, but the ICU is the safest place to be. Just in case . . ." My words and thoughts trailed off.

Mr. Herlan reached for my hand. "I'm kind of nervous, doctor. I don't really like hospitals and IVs and blood tests. Even Band-Aids give me the willies. Do you think you could call my friend John at home? Don't make it sound bad, but I'd like him to come to the hospital. Would you mind?" I nodded as we entered the ICU.

Six nurses descended like locusts upon Mr. Herlan. They whisked him from me and swallowed him into their domain, hooking him up with tubes, wires, and monitors. I leafed through the chart until I'd located John's number.

After the nurses finished mechanizing Mr. Herlan, it was the doctors' turn. Time to place the Swan-Ganz catheter into Mr. Herlan's body to monitor his internal pressures. Swans were much larger than standard central lines. Three feet of bright yellow rubber tubing that would loop from his jugular vein to his heart through to his lungs.

From there it would transmit detailed information about the blood pressure inside his heart and lungs.

I loved to show off to the interns how efficiently I could insert a Swan with barely any blood spilled from the needle stick. Then I'd impress them with the one-handed sutures I'd carefully honed over the years. Between the numerous Swans and central lines I'd done at Bellevue and my evening practice with mint dental floss, I could spin those one-handed sutures so dexterously that they appeared to arise like magic.

But this time, the Swan wouldn't go. I got my needle easily into the jugular vein, but I could not coax the catheter to float down to the heart. I wiggled the Swan, trying to take advantage of the natural curvature of the tubing, but it wouldn't go. I pulled back, then reinserted, but nothing happened. Just go in, damn it! I pushed and twisted and goaded and prayed. Come on, get in there! The bright yellow Swan curled up on the bedsheet mockingly. Two other people tried. The Swan would not yield.

I don't have time for this aggravation. I need to figure out what's going on with Mr. Herlan. I can't waste my energy with this stupid Swan. This isn't the ideal way to deal with a lactate of 6.8, but I can't get the damn thing in. I'll just have to live without those internal pressure readings.

"Because of initial technical difficulties placing a Swan-Ganz catheter, a regular central line was placed, along with a femoral arterial line."

Mr. Herlan's blood pressure hovered in the seventies. I couldn't let him sit with that low a pressure—any one of his organs could give out at any minute without sufficient blood and oxygen. Time to start pressors! I chewed on the edge of my tongue, hating to take such a drastic step without a Swan in place. Pressors without a Swan was like driving a car without a steering wheel, but there was no way around it. I had to get his blood pressure up.

"The patient was placed on a 'Neo' drip at eight P.M. The surgical resident recommended a gastrografin-swallow X-ray to evaluate for possible esophageal rupture."

I did another physical exam on Mr. Herlan, checking his heart and lungs. He did not have an "acute abdomen," suggesting an esophageal rupture, nor did he have a fever or elevated white count to suggest an infection. What the hell was going on? Why was his pressure dropping?

"I'm okay, really I am," Mr. Herlan said, his voice quivering faintly. "I just . . . just don't like X-rays, that's all. All that radiation and everything. Can't I just try some Mylanta? That's what John always gives me when I get like this, Mylanta and ginger ale. He says his grandmother swears by it." Mr. Herlan tried to laugh, but the sound came out in thin, stilted gasps. "I'm going to be okay, right?"

The gastrografin-swallow X-ray would show escaping dye if there was a rupture, but in order to do it I'd have to send him down to radiology on the second floor. Sending a patient out of the ICU with a tenuous blood pressure and a lactate of 6.8 was definitely courting disaster, but I needed to figure out what was going on. Otherwise, how would I be able to help him?

"The patient's blood pressure did not increase with maximum doses of Neo, therefore Levophed was added, again with minimal response."

"Another medicine, Doc? Do I really need another medicine?" Mr. Herlan asked as the nurses began the complicated process of preparing him for the trip down to X-ray. They arranged the many intravenous lines, the arterial line, the cardiac monitor, the blood pressure monitor, and the pulse oximeter on a portable cart. "What's going on, Doc? This is making me really nervous. I . . . I don't like all these medicines." His voice was beginning to sound parched.

I wished I knew what to tell him. "Well," I said, trying to sound casual, "your blood pressure is still a bit low. At this point it's not clear if it's an infection that is making you sick, or maybe a tiny hole from the balloon. If this special X-ray shows a hole then the surgeons would come to fix it." No big deal, just a lactate of 6.8 that I can't explain. Just a crashing patient that I have no clue about.

"Surgeons? An operation? I don't know about that, Doc." Sweat was accumulating at his hairline. "I'm really feeling scared, Doc.

Really scared. Do you think you could give me something to calm down? Just a little something, because I . . . I get nervous in situations like this."

I hesitated, not wanting to further complicate an already confusing situation. "It wouldn't be the best idea, because it could lower your blood pressure, and it's already pretty low. I'd like to avoid making things worse."

"Please Doc. You gotta help me." Mr. Herlan grabbed my hand forcefully and pulled himself up. There was a wild look in his eyes. "Please, I'm not going to make it otherwise. I'm really, really scared. Hospitals always make me scared."

Medically, I thought it was the wrong thing to do. What if I made him worse? I had to watch out for myself, too. Mr. Herlan looked at me beseechingly. His words were coming in fits and starts. "Please Doc. I get anxiety attacks. Ask John, he knows . . . especially when I'm in hospitals. I get so scared." His hair was plastered to his forehead with sweat and his pupils were as wide as cat's eyes.

But how could I leave him in this state? The poor guy was terrified. I asked the nurse for a tiny dose of a sedative, hoping for a placebo effect. Before I injected it, I sent off an arterial blood gas to check his oxygen status.

"At nine P.M. the patient was being readied to go to radiology, but his blood pressure was still low and he was complaining of increased anxiety. A blood gas was sent and 0.5 mg of IV midazolam was administered."

Predictably, the sedative did nothing. Placebos rarely work when you really need them. Mr. Herlan became more and more agitated. He was twisting in bed trying to sit up. "You gotta help me, Doc. Give me something more." He yanked at my white coat, his teeth chattering. "I'm so scared." He was breathing heavily and panting out his words. "I can't take it anymore," he sputtered. "I'm really scared!" This was about to be a disaster—I didn't need the results of the blood gas to know.

"Intubate this man right now," I snapped, "he's about to go

down!" The nurses rushed over with equipment trays. I was ready to do it myself, but Mr. Herlan was a lot more agitated than Leo Teitelbaum had been when I did my very first intubation. Mr. Herlan was awake and fighting, whereas Mr. Teitelbaum had coded and was unconscious—or dead, depending on how you looked at it. Luckily the anesthesiologist arrived quickly. He placed the laryngoscope in Mr. Herlan's mouth and started to feed in the breathing tube, but Mr. Herlan jerked his head violently and threw his elbows into the air. He coughed and gasped for breath, lashing out with his arms. I tried to explain why we had to do this, but he clawed desperately at us. I held him down and rubbed his chest with my palm while the anesthesiologist took a break from trying to force down the tube. He clamped an oxygen mask over Mr. Herlan's face and took a few breaths himself. I was glad I wasn't doing the intubation.

"Listen to me," I said, trying to make my voice sound calm and reassuring. "I know this is horrible, but you need this tube to breathe." Alarms were squawking and the oxygen mask was fogging up around Mr. Herlan's mouth and nose. "It's uncomfortable going in, but it's going to make you breathe better. You've got to trust me." Mr. Herlan continued to thrash. Tears were running into his oxygen mask and they sloshed recklessly each time he swung his head. Reluctantly, I turned to the anesthesiologist. "Put him out."

"The patient was intubated with some difficulty at nine forty-five P.M. on Saturday night. Heavy sedation was required. Copious pink frothy sputum was noted in the endotracheal tube."

"Shit," I said, "he's in pulmonary edema. His lungs have flooded. Twenty milligrams of IV Lasix, stat!" I shouted. "Somebody get me an EKG machine!"

"The EKG showed sinus tachycardia with normal intervals, but there were no R waves. The admission EKG had been normal."

"What the hell is going on now?" Panic started to constrict my stomach. "Is he having an MI?" I asked to no one in particular. "He's too young for a heart attack! He's only thirty-one. Get me another Swan-Ganz catheter kit. I've got to get a Swan in."

*Just stay calm. Stay calm. Gotta get that Swan in to figure out
what's going on inside. Don't puncture the lung when the needle goes
in. You still have a clean record in the pneumothorax department.
Residency is over in a couple of months—this isn't the time to drop
a lung. Just stay calm. Don't drip sweat on the sterile field. Ease that
needle into the jugular. Don't let your hands shake.*

*Good blood return, now slide in the guide wire, nice and easy.
Don't cause any arrythmias when you get near the heart. Don't
puncture any vessels. Now ease that catheter in. Slow and steady.
Your patient is crashing, but you gotta stay calm and focus on the
Swan going in. If you screw up now you could really make things
worse. Right atrium, right ventricle, pulmonary artery. Wedge the
balloon, slow and steady, don't cause a pulmonary hemorrhage . . .
and we're in.*

Thank you, God.

"Initial Swan-Ganz readings were: pulmonary artery pressures of
48/39, wedge pressure of 42, cardiac output of 3.6. Patient continued to
produce pink, frothy sputum."

*Jesus, he's in cardiogenic shock, his whole circulatory system is col-
lapsing. I think I'm collapsing. What the hell is going on?*

*Everything was happening so fast that I hadn't even thought
about calling the GI attending. This is UH, I reminded myself—I
have to call the attending. And it's not even Mr. Herlan's regular
doctor, it's a covering attending.*

*I stumbled over my breaths as I recounted the downward spiral of
the evening over the phone. I prayed that the attending would have
some magical solution that I hadn't thought of. After all, he was the
attending. But he didn't. I asked him for permission to obtain a cardiology consult and a critical care consult.*

*The intern leaned over my shoulder, "Is the attending going to
come in tonight?"*

*"Nope," I said. "He didn't even offer. Thinks we're doing a great
job, though." Life in a private hospital. Only a few more months of
being at the bottom of the heap.*

I called the critical care attending at home. Maybe he would be so impressed by the gravity of the situation that he would drop his Saturday night plans and come right over to the hospital. But he didn't. I know, it's a hassle driving in from Westchester. He suggested that we evaluate for auto-peep on the ventilator. The cardiology attending didn't offer to see the patient either; he sent over the cardiology fellow instead.

"The blood gas revealed severe acidosis, with a pH of 7.0."

Bicarb," I shouted, my voice starting to crack. "I need bicarb." If his pH drops any further, he's going to code any minute now. "Two amps of bicarb, stat!"

Mr. Herlan was bucking the vent and thrashing in bed. He fought the air that was pulsing down his throat. Additional sedatives weren't helping. Cardiogenic shock, severe acidosis, and I can't even get him to take in the oxygen that he needs. "Let's start a pancuronium drip," I called out to the nurse. It was a last ditch effort, but paralyzing all his muscles might be the only way to allow the ventilator to give him oxygen. I wasn't going to waste time calling the required pulmonary consult for this one.

The nurse pointed out his blood pressure. It was in the 60s even with the Neo and the Levophed running in at maximum doses.

Damn! What else to do? Think of something. Anything. Now.

"Dobutamine! Let's get a dobutamine drip going." I didn't know what the hell a third pressor would do if the first two hadn't worked, but I had to do something. "Another round of Lasix, IV push! Let's go."

Stay calm. Keep thinking. Hypotension. Cardiogenic shock. Pulmonary edema. Severe acidosis. What's the common factor? Which is the cause and which is the effect? What's precipitating the whole chain of events? Think, damn it. Think.

The nurses buzzed furiously at Mr. Herlan's bedside administering the medications. All the patients in the ICU were watching the action at Mr. Herlan's bed. I stood in the middle pressing my hands against my temples trying to make the brain cells work harder. Think, damn it. Think.

In the meantime, Mr. Herlan's friend John had arrived. I didn't want him to see all that was going on at the bedside so I took him to the ICU lounge. How to say that the patient is crashing and the doctors don't have a clue. The words ensnarled my tongue, mocking my frustration and ignorance. I wanted to scream, I wanted to vomit. I wanted to curl up in a corner and make Mr. Herlan, the oppressive ICU, the damn Swan-Ganz catheter, and the paralyzing pancuronium drip all disappear. But I sputtered out some vague words about "hovering blood pressure" and "possible infection." John listened attentively and waited politely for me to finish. Then he spoke.

"Raphael and I have been together for more than five years. I've seen him go through lots of hard times. When he tried to kill himself three years ago, that was the worst. But he's gotten a lot better and we've had some very happy times. One thing I know is that he doesn't want to suffer. Do what you can, Doctor, but if it seems like you can't save him, let him go. Just don't let him be in pain. I promised him that I would always look out for him. Please . . ."

I led John to the ICU for a quick visit. Mr. Herlan's skin was ashen but his body was now calm. John could not know that the stillness was a cruel pharmaceutical hoax from the pancuronium. I stared at the preternaturally tranquil body. What was raging inside? What was the answer? John held Mr. Herlan's hand and spoke quietly to him for a few minutes. The nurse tapped him gently and said it was time to go.

"The cardiology fellow arrived at eleven-thirty P.M. on Saturday night. A bedside echocardiogram revealed diffuse left ventricular hypokinesis. The cardiology attending was consulted by phone. He felt that the cardiogenic shock was likely secondary to esophageal rupture, not to a primary process in the heart. Therefore neither an aortic balloon pump nor an emergent cardiac angiogram were indicated.

"At that point the patient's blood pressure was 64/35 on max doses of Neo, Levo, and dobutamine. Pink, frothy sputum continued to accumulate in the endotracheal tube despite vigorous and repeated suctioning. Over the next few hours the pressure slipped to 43/27."

I called back the GI attending. His voice was heavy from slum-

ber. He reminded me again that he was only covering. "Listen," I pleaded, "this patient is going down the tubes despite everything I am doing. He's in cardiogenic shock, but cardiology doesn't want to get involved because they don't think it's a primary cardiac problem. Surgery doesn't want to get involved because he doesn't have an acute abdomen."

I felt my voice beginning to break. "Surgery wants a gastrografin-swallow X-ray, but he's too unstable to send down to radiology. I'm trying to convince the surgeons to take him to the OR anyway to look for a ruptured esophagus, but they won't take him with a blood pressure of 43/27. The critical care consult won't come in to the hospital."

Please, please don't let me start crying on the phone. "I'm treating him with triple antibiotics even though he has no signs of infection. He's on three pressors but his blood pressure is still bottoming out. I even had to paralyze his body just so I could get some oxygen in him. I don't know what else to do!"

"At two A.M. the covering GI attending came in to the hospital. All the X-rays in the patient's folder were reviewed."

We arranged the X-rays in chronological order. The GI attending, the surgery resident, the intern, and I examined each and every film. We scrutinized them for "free air" that would indicate esophageal rupture. Each chest X-ray showed a line of clearing just behind the heart. We all agreed that it wasn't free air—it was just an unusual shadow resulting from the surgically attached piece of colon where his esophagus had been repaired. We pored over every lab result and every Swan-Ganz reading. We listened to Mr. Herlan's lungs and palpated his abdomen.

The attending sighed and looked at the three of us. "I don't have the answer, either. You guys have done an excellent job, but I think it's over now. Just keep him comfortable." He turned to me, "Listen, since you know Mr. Herlan's friend and I've never met him, would you mind explaining all this to him?" I nodded my head numbly, too weary to argue about whose responsibility the "discussion" should be. The attending jotted a note in the chart and went home. It was nearly four A.M.

"At that point the decision was made for supportive care only."

I went into the lounge to find John. "I've called Raphael's parents," he said as I walked in. "They're catching the next plane in from St. Louis."

I recounted the events of the night. He nodded gravely with each pronouncement that I made. I finally led up to the inevitable. "At this point," I hesitated, hating my job, hating the attending, "I think there is not much more we can do." I gestured stupidly in the air, batting at my meager words. "We'll just have to watch and wait. But we'll make sure that he is comfortable."

John didn't blink. "I understand, Doctor, and I appreciate your efforts. I just don't want him to be in any pain. Would it ... would it be okay if I spent a few hours with him? Just until morning?"

I accompanied John to the ICU, but when I saw Mr. Herlan, I had John wait at the door. I asked the nurse to help me.

The nurse and I moved the EKG machine away from Mr. Herlan's bed. We unhooked a few IVs that were not necessary. We tucked extraneous wires and tubes behind the bed. We covered the yellow Swan-Ganz catheter sticking out of his neck with a folded white pillowcase. We removed the old bandages and cleaned his skin where there were sticky traces of surgical tape. We switched the blood pressure and oxygen monitors from his arms down to his legs so that the blanket would hide them. We adjusted the breathing tube in his mouth so the saliva wouldn't accumulate in the corners. We swept away the extra syringes and gauze pads from his windowsill. We changed his hospital gown and combed his hair. Then I called John in.

From the door I watched John clasp Mr. Herlan's hand in his own and kneel at the bedside. He rested his head on their interlocked fingers.

"The patient's friend remained at the bedside for the duration of the night."

Dawn broke only a few hours later. The sedatives and paralytics were slowly wearing off. John came out to tell us that he thought Raphael was responding to him. We all crowded at the bedside in disbelief, but indeed Mr. Herlan responded to the simple commands of "Squeeze my hand" and "Open your eyes." A chill ran through my shoulders and my palms flew to my mouth. Faint rays of sunlight filtered over the gray of the East River and trickled into the ICU. There was magic to a new day, I knew it all along. I held my face tight, afraid that a smile might jinx our good luck. Mr. Herlan's blood pressure was still 54/34 on maximum doses of three pressors, and his lactate was still high, but he was responsive! His brain was somehow still getting oxygen. Silently I cheered for the sun. I rooted for it to climb high and dazzle its brilliance into our little corner of the ICU. I dispatched the intern to call the attending. "I don't care what time it is. Wake him up."

"The covering GI attending was contacted and informed of the patient's condition. He felt we should continue with supportive care only."

"What? He doesn't want us to do anything else?"

The intern nodded silently at me.

"Jesus Christ! I hate this place." I started pacing violently in the cramped workspace of the ICU. "I mean, the patient is still in terrible shape, but at least he's somewhat responsive now. That's more than we had five hours ago." I banged into the chart rack each time I whirled around. There was clattering as vials of saline flipped over onto the floor. "I don't know what else to do, but we have to do something! Get critical care on the phone."

"The critical care attending was also contacted. He suggested an epinephrine drip, but said he would not be in the hospital that day."

Now it was Sunday. My thirty hours were over. I was reluctant to go home and let anyone else take care of Mr. Herlan, but I had no choice. I slept fitfully during the day, calling the ICU every few hours. There was no change in Mr. Herlan's condition.

First thing Monday morning I sprinted over to the hospital, even before I had my coffee. Mr. Herlan was already dead. I grabbed the chart and the intern and demanded to know what had happened.

The intern was despondent. I could see the exhaustion in his body as he labored to speak. "Sunday morning Mr. Herlan was really responsive to me. He nodded his head and squeezed my hand to answer my questions. I kept trying to convince the attending to get another cardiology consult but he wouldn't do it. He just wanted to stick with supportive care."

The intern rubbed his eyes and then reached for a 10cc syringe. "Another cardiologist was in the ICU visiting a different patient," he continued, pulling and pushing on the plunger of the syringe, "and I asked him to take a look at Mr. Herlan. He didn't want to get involved unless he was officially consulted. But I pleaded with him, I begged him until he finally said yes."

"The patient was seen by a different cardiology attending on Sunday whose impression was 'cardiogenic shock with acute myocardial infarction superimposed on underlying cardiomyopathy.'"

"So he agreed with us," I said, "that Mr. Herlan was having a heart attack."

"Yeah," sighed the intern, "but he couldn't say if it was the primary event, or just secondary to either esophageal rupture or overwhelming infection. Besides, Mr. Herlan was too unstable at that point for any cardiac intervention, so there was nothing the cardiologist could do. Mr. Herlan's blood pressure was so low, but somehow his brain was still working. He was communicating with me, I swear he was. He heard my words." The intern looked at me with heavy eyes.

"Sunday morning the patient's family and significant other made him DNR. Over the next twelve hours the patient's blood pressure remained at 40/20 and he gradually became less responsive."

I dropped the chart and stormed into the chief resident's office. "You'll never believe this case from the weekend," I burst out. "I don't know what the hell went wrong!"

My chief resident looked up at me blandly from the journal she was reading. "Oh, Mr. Herlan? He had free air in his heart. That's why he went into cardiogenic shock and died."

"Free air?" My muscles froze. "What free air? When did he have free air in his heart?"

She looked at me, half-bored, half-incredulous, "On Friday afternoon, right after the balloon procedure. It's in the X-ray report. Didn't you read it?"

I reached for the edge of the desk for support. I could feel my blood pressure plummeting as the chief resident calmly scrolled through the X-ray reports on her computer screen. "It's right here—'Free air superimposed in the right heart and base of the aorta, most likely within the pericardium or anterior mediastinum.'"

I sank back into the chair, my head reeling. Could I have missed that? Did I not notice free air? I had examined every single X-ray myself.

But I hadn't, I realized with rising nausea, read the written X-ray reports.

Usually the radiologists call immediately if they see an "emergency" problem. As the clinician, however, it was still my responsibility to read the X-ray reports in addition to examining the actual X-rays. It wasn't the radiologist's fault, it was mine. I killed Mr. Herlan.

"Family and significant other remained at the bedside. Patient became asystolic and was pronounced dead at twelve thirty-five P.M."

I stumbled over the final words, trying vainly to keep my voice from cracking. I took a sip of my lukewarm coffee. I closed my presentation by quoting the X-ray report:

"Free air superimposed in the right heart and base of the aorta, most likely within the pericardium or mediastinum."

I lowered my eyes, adding that I had only read these reports on Monday morning, after the patient had died.

My words fell off into an aching silence.

Was I supposed to say something else?

The head of the department turned to the radiologist and asked her to formally review the X-rays. She, herself, was only a moonlighter, who had been covering for someone else that weekend.

The radiologist pointed to the X-ray that had been taken just after the balloon procedure on Friday. With a sober, Eastern European accent, she explained the findings. "Here we can see some air next to the heart. I reported it as being within the pericardium or the mediastinum." Her voice began to quiver. "I should have called the doctors immediately. I should have, I know." She was nearly whispering. "But I did not. I made a mistake."

I tried to swallow, but my tongue was caked to the roof of my mouth. The heavy air of the room seemed to shrink around me, pressing on my eardrums with that horrible feeling like a plane plunging downward toward unforgiving concrete.

The radiologist paused, attempting to smooth her white coat with trembling fingers. Her hands skittered off the stiff material and hung, twitching, in the air. "But now I realize that I had made two mistakes. This is not free air in the heart," she stammered. "It's not free air at all; it's only a shadow from the piece of colon that was added during his surgery three years ago." She swallowed, and then her voice petered out to a whisper. "This X-ray is normal."

The room was silent. The radiologist slumped down in her chair and her head collapsed into her hands. I tried to breathe a sigh of relief, but my mouth was too dry. My eardrums were still throbbing.

The head of the department opened up the case for discussion. Most of the audience members stared down at their fingers. One or two spoke up with some irrelevant comments on minor details. A few glared at me from across the room. No spirited academic debate ensued. No enlightened educational themes emerged. The proceedings were conspicuously anemic.

I wanted to get up and scream. I wanted to yell at these pompous attendings who had abandoned the patient and the residents. I had called them at home. I had pleaded with them for help.

This is supposed to be a teaching institution, I wanted to holler. I am still a doctor-in-training. Where were they that night?

And what about collegial respect, I wanted to add. The patient's well-being notwithstanding, why couldn't they have risen to the occasion for my sake? I was crashing on that night also. Couldn't they have helped me? We're all on the same team, aren't we? We're supposed to be colleagues, right?

But I said nothing. I still had to deal with these attendings in the future.

If this patient had been at Bellevue instead of UH, I wanted to shout in their faces, it all would have been different. The residents, not the attendings, would have been in charge. We wouldn't have had to beg for a cardiology consult. This patient would at least have been taken to the OR to look for an esophageal rupture before his blood pressure had bottomed out.

But no, in this place we were not allowed to make any decisions without the attendings' permission, the same attendings who wouldn't get out of bed to see the damn patient. They didn't have to sit with the patient's friend at four in the morning and confess that our fancy medicines and high-tech ICU were powerless. They didn't have to watch the patient's lover kneeling at the bedside for hours. They didn't have to look at the patient squeezing John's hand, and then spit out someone else's opinion that the situation was hopeless, even though there might still have been a chance. They didn't have to witness a patient their own age slowly expire before their eyes while they stood by like a useless shaman.

I remained silent. The truth was, I realized miserably, no matter what we might have done, Mr. Herlan would probably have died anyway.

The preliminary autopsy report was read aloud. There was no perforation of the esophagus. No bacteria were identified in his blood. No traces of illicit drugs were found.

The department head felt that the cause of death was most likely from widespread infection, despite the fact that the bacterial cultures were negative. Micro-perforations from the balloon had probably released intestinal bacteria into the bloodstream. The resultant infection overwhelmed the heart and circulatory system.

"In reality," the department head concluded, "Mr. Herlan died of his own hand. It took three years for his suicide attempt to be completed, but it finally killed him."

I sat in my chair as the conference room emptied, my limbs unable to respond to my commands for their movement. The critical care attending came over to point out that I had never specifically asked him to come in to the hospital that night. I could only look at him blankly.

The room was shrinking around me fast. My eardrums felt like they were about to implode from the pressure. My stomach was in knots and the taste of vomit was in my mouth. I suddenly had an overwhelming urge to disembowel someone with my own bare hands.

But I just didn't know who.

CHAPTER FOURTEEN

Intensive Care

They cannot scare me with their empty spaces
Between stars—on stars where no human race is.
I have it in me so much nearer home
To scare myself with my own desert places.

Robert Frost, "Desert Places"

THE PATIENT WAS A routine alcoholic, hauled off the streets of Manhattan on a warm June evening and brought to the Bellevue emergency room. Or maybe he staggered into the ER. In either case, when his dose of Thunderbird or Mad Dog wore off, he slid into alcohol withdrawal. The ER staff probably gave him ten milligrams of Valium to stop the shakes and racing heart rate. Then twenty milligrams, then forty. Apparently they'd been unable to calm the tremors and agitation at even the highest doses of Valium and so started giving him barbiturates—the "big guns." Eventually they did silence his tremors, and in the process, his breathing. So by the time he arrived in our ICU, he was intubated with a breathing tube down his throat and a heaving ventilator at his side pushing in the oxygen. There was nothing else to do except wait out the days until the barbiturates wore off so we could extubate him and allow him to breathe on his own.

Now we stood in front of our patient in Bed 12, his disheveled street looks frozen in place by the barbiturate coma. Lauren was presenting the case. She was a shy, petite intern with a mousy demeanor. Dr. Sitkin, our lanky six-foot attending, slouched against the IV pole as she spoke, a derisive half-smile on his face the entire time. He shook his head slowly when she finally finished. "Jeez," he said, in his Tennessee drawl, "where do they unearth these ER docs? Haven't they ever read a textbook in their lives, or do they still use garlic cloves down there?"

Lauren reddened and looked down quickly. "I'm serious now," Dr. Sitkin said, standing up and straightening out the slight hunch of his shoulders. "It's like hauling in a John Deere tractor to knock off a pesky moth. Now this guy ain't gonna be whistling Dixie for some time.

"What day is it today, anyway?" He glanced down at his watch. "June third? This guy ain't gonna wake up this week." His hands began to gesticulate in the air. "This guy ain't gonna wake up this month. Or next month. This guy ain't gonna wake up until at least Rosh Hashana." He pointed to the ventilator. "In fact, why don't we just park a shofar on this ol' ventilator. When he starts blowing the shofar, we'll know it's time to extubate him."

I didn't want to do it. I didn't want to laugh in front of a patient. I didn't want to laugh at a patient. Again. But the image of our homeless alcoholic blowing the ram's horn in Bed 12 of the ICU just rocked my funny bone, and to my embarrassment and annoyance, I once again found myself laughing uncontrollably on rounds with Dr. Sitkin. I thought his humor was off-color, inappropriate, and sometimes downright insulting to the patients and the staff. But the combination of his dry Jewish humor and his Southern drawl just overpowered my self-control. In between his jokes he freely peppered us with educational pearls. His breadth of knowledge extended way beyond his field of infectious disease—he was always impressing us with arcane fungi and protozoa—to all of general internal medicine and critical care medicine. But he was equally free with his biting criticism for anyone who wasn't as smart or as fast as he, which was most of the world.

Dr. Sitkin looked around at our team, which was a healthy mix of ethnicities and colors. His lean face screwed up in a smirk and his bushel of wiry salt-and-pepper hair cascaded over his brow. He eased his tiny wire-rimmed glasses low down on his bony nose and his eyes darted over the tops. "For the *goyim* amongst us, there's a copy of the Talmud in my office next to my other bible, *Mandel's Infectious Disease*. You can consult either one if you need a refresher on Rosh Hashana ritual." He shoved his glasses back up and sauntered on to the next patient.

"This one's dead," he said passing by my patient with metastatic esophageal cancer in Bed 11. "What's he doing in our ICU?"

"His daughter hasn't signed the DNR yet," I said.

"Rubbish. There's no rule about having to administer critical care to a corpse just because there's no DNR in place. You don't have to give medical care that's not warranted. Ship this guy out." On Dr. Sitkin marched and our team jogged to catch up with his long strides.

"Dead. Dead. Dead," he pronounced, moving swiftly past the Alzheimer's patient with three strokes in Bed 10, the woman with metastatic lung cancer in Bed 9, and the demented bilateral amputee with renal failure and liver failure in Bed 8. On the days when our other attending, Dr. Marks, rounded with us, we spent a full ten minutes at each bedside reviewing the labs, the X-rays, and the medications. The poor prognosis would be acknowledged in an oblique way, but the entire treatment plan would be discussed and debated as with any other patient. Only Dr. Sitkin had the honesty—or the chutzpah, depending on your viewpoint—to call it like it was. "Dead. Dead. Dead. Why are we wasting our time even talking?" The team would shuffle along uncomfortably, knowing that he was right in a way—all these patients were going to die in the near future no matter what we did—but it didn't seem proper, somehow, to say that right out in the open.

Bed 11—"Dead." Bed 10—"Dead." Bed 9—"Dead." Bed 8—"Dead."

Bed 7. This was where Dr. Sitkin would stop. Stop walking and stop joking. Li-Feng Chen was thirty-two years old. Her leukemia had been in remission for two years, but six months into her pregnancy it flared up with a "blast crisis." Determined to keep her baby, she avoided chemotherapy until she was so sick that she required an emergency Caesarian section. The baby was downstairs in the neonatal ICU; Ms. Chen was upstairs in the adult ICU. Her bone marrow had been devastated by the leukemia and her body was now a veritable Petri dish for infection.

"This is a patient who deserves our ICU," Dr. Sitkin said. "This is a patient who might be able to benefit from our intensive monitoring." On the days we rounded with Dr. Sitkin, we spent 98 percent of our time in front of Ms. Chen's bed. He demanded to know every lab value, the exact dose of every medication, the specific chemotherapy regimen. He'd perch on the edge of the chart rack and grill us on the minutiae of her care. And then he'd scrunch up his face and think. Minutes of silence would follow as the whole team watched him cogitate. He'd rub his nonexistent beard or twirl the wedding ring around his finger. Then he'd say, "I'm not satisfied with her antibiotic coverage. She's at risk both from typical infections seen in oncology patients as well as those from a gynecological source. Let's start from scratch." He'd have us draw more blood cultures, repeat a spinal tap, change all of her IV lines, and then start her on new antibiotics.

On the railing of Ms. Chen's bed was a Polaroid picture of her baby. It was a scrawny thing with a full head of wet black hair, sporting nearly as many tubes and catheters as her mother. As we left Bed 7, I always thought I caught Dr. Sitkin stealing a glance at that photo.

Dr. Sitkin was not shy about sharing with us the latest exploits of Andrea, his eight-month-old. "Yesterday she discovered her toes," he announced during a conference. "Don't ask me how she did it, but she managed to get all five of her toes in her mouth at once. The kid's a genius. My wife and I attempted the same thing, and I warn you . . . don't try this at home without the proper safety mechanisms."

One day I had to choose which antibiotics to give to my patient with metastatic esophageal cancer after he had spiked a new fever. I debated which combination of drugs I should use and then I thought, "Gee, we have a specialist in infectious diseases this month, let me give him a call." I left a message at Dr. Sitkin's private practice office and he called back promptly. I described the situation and asked his advice.

"My advice is that you grow up and make your own decisions. Don't page me to choose some designer assortment of antibiotics. I don't care which ones you use, the patient's dead anyway." He hung up the phone and I felt ashamed of my juvenile question.

Every Wednesday we had "ICU touchy-feely rounds." One of the psychiatrists met with the residents over a pizza lunch to discuss any feelings we had about our time in the ICU. Our attendings were deliberately not present so we could feel free to talk. Frequently, we bitched about the long hours. Occasionally someone talked about a difficult

patient. But mostly we complained about Dr. Sitkin. About how inap
propriate he could be. About his constant jokes at the expense of pa
tients. About how we were made to be "colluders" in his humor. About
how he had no patience for 95 percent of the staff and 95 percent of the
patients. About how we were nervous presenting cases in front of him
because he always had cutting criticism to offer.

On Wednesday afternoons he'd catch my eye with a wink and say
"Did you all have a good time kvetching about me?" I would smil
sheepishly and he'd say, "That's okay. All of your complaints are prob
ably justified—I'm a boor, I'm insensitive, I'm condescending."

I'd nod cautiously. "Well, a few things like that were mentioned."

"Good, good," he'd smile. "It's heartening to know that I'm not lo
ing my touch."

I decided to take a risk and push a little bit. "Well some people fe
a little uncomfortable with all the jokes, Dr. Sitkin."

"Jokes? Every goddamn person here is dying. What else can you d
but joke? You guys take everything so seriously. Relax a little."

"Some people are a little uncomfortable during the case presenta
tions because you come down so hard on them."

He shook his head in disbelief. "Listen, I'm never going to lie to an
one. You can trust me on that. Whaddya guys want, a goddamn kinde
garten ice cream party?"

I shrugged. "That wouldn't be so bad."

The next day during conference Dr. Sitkin hauled in twelve pints
Ben & Jerry's ice cream. "Ofri thinks I'm being too harsh on you
he announced, plunking them on the table one by one, their lids gli
tening with frost. "She thinks I should get you some ice cream to mak
you feel better." The room was silent for a moment. But residents a
residents and free food is free food, even if it was ice cream for brea
fast. Everyone dove in with their plastic spoons, competing for t
good flavors like Chocolate Chip Cookie Dough and NY Super Fud
Chunk.

Dr. Sitkin licked a spoonful of vanilla. "How am I doing, Ofri?"
asked dryly. "Better?"

. . .

❧During our case conference the following week, Lauren was presenting one of the admissions from the previous night. Lauren could have passed for twelve years old. Everything about her—her wispy voice, her four-foot-ten height, her shyness, her wide, innocent eyes—appeared childlike. Dr. Sitkin's raucous sarcasm made her visibly nervous. Even though she'd grown up on the same side of the Mason-Dixon Line as he, she'd inherited the more genteel aspects of Southernism, while Dr. Sitkin was more of a Brooklynite cloaked in a Tennessee drawl.

Lauren read from her admission note. The note was long and overly detailed. Lauren's nervousness kept her from even once looking up from the printed page. She labored over word after word, too tense to include any inflection or pause. Even I couldn't deny that it was boring as she plodded along. We all were feeling the somnolent effects of her dry presentation and struggled to stay focused. Dr. Sitkin rolled his eyes. Then he rolled his neck, loudly cracking a joint. Then he plunked his head on the table and left it there, curled up in his arms.

We sat in stunned silence. Slowly we looked from one to the other. We'd never seen an attending do that before; nobody knew what to do. Lauren resumed reading from her admission note in a tentative voice, but Dr. Sitkin didn't stir. Eventually her voice petered out and we sat riveted to our seats.

No one said or did anything to break the silence. Finally I took a deep breath. "Should we call a code?" I asked.

Smiles bubbled up on people's faces, but no one wanted to laugh out loud. Dr. Sitkin snapped his head upward and the team giggled, then burst out laughing. He looked at me and I wasn't sure if it was a look of anger or humor. He nodded slowly. "Good one Ofri. Touché."

❧Ms. Chen grew sicker. Her leukemia had spun out of control, taking her immune system with it; the infections were getting the best of her. Every morning on rounds, we sped through the ICU until Dr. Sitkin parked us at Bed 7. We plowed through the data exhaustively, hunting for a chink in the relentless progression of her pathology through which we could intervene. "Leukemia can be a curable disease," Dr. Sitkin insisted. "If we can pull her through this crisis, she still might achieve a remission, if not a permanent cure. Forget all the corpses in the other beds; this is where our attention should be."

The nurses from the neonatal ICU paid visits frequently to update Ms. Chen on her daughter's condition. Ms. Chen had not seen her daughter since the birth four weeks ago. She'd had a few minutes to meet her baby in the delivery room before each was whisked to her respective ICU. The Polaroids on the railing were updated weekly.

When Ms. Chen began to bleed from her gut we transfused her. When she began to have seizures we hauled her and all of her machinery downstairs for a head CT. When her lungs weakened we intubated her and gave her a breathing tube.

"I only give up when there's no hope," Dr. Sitkin said. "And there's still hope." He still made "whale blubber" remarks about the obese demented lady in Bed 2. He still had no patience for the end-stage AIDS patient in Bed 3, even though a large portion of his private practice consisted of AIDS patients. "I have nothing against dying—it's a noble process—but it should be done at home or in a regular medical bed. Not in the ICU. This is the place to give intensive care when there is a possibility of meaningful recovery. We're not a hospice here."

On that Tuesday morning when we told him that Ms. Chen had died overnight, Dr. Sitkin was quiet and only nodded. He asked us to tell him in detail what had happened. We described the incessant hemorrhaging and intractable fevers. We described the bottoming blood pressure that refused to respond to any intervention. We told him how her lungs flooded despite the forced air of the ventilator. We told him how her seizures continued unabated. We told him that we pronounced her dead at 4:53 A.M. and then called her family. He nodded throughout. "Good job," he said at the end, his voice uncharacteristically soft. "You guys did a good job."

℘On the last day of our month in the ICU, we sat with Dr. Sitkin in the conference room. "Okay guys, here's your chance to tell me what you think of me. We're going around the room in ascending order of seniority—interns first. Be brutally honest, because that's how I'd be with you. And don't worry—anything you say today has probably been said before about me."

He pointed to Lauren. "You first."

Lauren immediately reddened.

"C'mon Lauren. Lay it on the line. I ain't made of glass," he drawled.

Lauren cleared her throat. "Well, I appreciated all the stuff you taught us about infectious disease."

"Don't worry, you don't have to make me feel good."

"Well sometimes you made me feel shy. You made me feel like I couldn't do anything good."

Dr. Sitkin nodded and twirled his wedding ring. "Good, good, now we're getting somewhere. Keep it coming."

"But I can do things good," she said.

"Tell me, Lauren. What can you do good?"

She paused. "I can sing."

"Sing?"

"Yes, I sing every Sunday in church."

Dr. Sitkin smiled and leaned back in his chair. "By all means, Lauren. Sing us a song."

Lauren looked at him, confused.

"I'm serious," Dr. Sitkin said. "Sing us a song."

Lauren adjusted her lab coat then stood up slowly. She focused on a spot over our heads and opened her mouth. Out came the loudest, clearest soprano that I'd ever heard. All of her diffidence and "childlikeness" suddenly melted away. It was as though when she stood up those robes slipped away onto the chair behind her. She belted out a church hymn that was almost too powerful for our little conference room. We were jolted awake and mesmerized by this stunning, compelling woman before us. When she finished, she sat down abruptly.

Dr. Sitkin was visibly moved. "Thank you Lauren. I have to say that's never happened to me before." Back in her seat, Lauren was as physically diminutive as she'd always been, but she never again appeared childlike to me.

Dr. Sitkin went around the room pointing at each intern and then each resident who gave him some feedback. When he got to me, he went out of order and skipped to the pulmonary fellow who was actually above me in seniority. "You're last Ofri. I'm saving the best for last."

When it was finally my turn the room quieted. Everyone seemed to expect a face-off because they knew I had criticized him heavily both in person and in "touchy-feely rounds."

"Well, Sitkin," I said. "This month has been nothing if not interesting. You have been a unique attending in all my time at Bellevue. I appreciate your honesty and I know that you really do care about the patients and us, even if you won't always admit to it." I took a deep breath. "But at times you are entirely inappropriate, juvenile, insulting, and downright nasty. I sometimes can't believe that the department lets you run free like this, entrusting the education of impressionable young interns to you. And I hate the way you make fun of sick patients who are dying. I think that's despicable."

"Whew," Dr. Sitkin said. "I was worried for a moment that you were actually going to say something bad about me."

"The worst thing is," I continued, "is that I find your disgusting humor incredibly funny and I've actually enjoyed this month in the ICU."

"Praise the Lord," he said, looking upward. "She likes me. Ofri actually likes me."

I had been visiting a friend at the beach on Long Island one weekend in early August and biked over to the Amagansett Farmers' Market to pick up some bagels. Sitting on one of the wooden benches by a bin of freshly harvested corn was Dr. Sitkin and his wife. A racing bike leaned against the back of the bench. When he saw me, he smiled and beckoned me over.

"Julie," he said to his wife, "this is Danielle Ofri, one of the best residents from Bellevue."

A compliment from Sitkin? An honest-to-goodness compliment? It took me a moment to absorb what he'd just said and then I could feel a goofy grin spread from ear to ear, but I couldn't help it. A compliment from Sitkin. When I recovered from my shock I reached out and shook hands with his wife. "It's a pleasure to meet you. Your husband is a one-of-a-kind attending."

Julie smiled. "He certainly is a one-of-a-kind guy. And you must be a one-of-a-kind resident if you managed to survive with him and still come out smiling."

"We actually had a lot of fun in the ICU," I said. "Do you come out here often?"

"We have a house here in East Hampton," Julie said. "Most weekends we're here, though Joseph spends more time on his bike than in the house."

"That's not true," Dr. Sitkin said in mock protest. "Just once a day I take a spin to Sag Harbor to stretch my legs." East Hampton to Sag Harbor was twenty miles round-trip and it wasn't all flat.

"Hey Ofri," Dr. Sitkin said, "you haven't met the most important members of the family." He lifted a baby out of the stroller that was parked next to the bench. "This little sweetheart is Andrea." He cradled her in his arms and tickled her chin so she would smile at me.

"Ah, yes, the one who can get all her toes in her mouth."

"Precisely. And the real genius of the family is Ellen. Ellen? Where are you hiding?"

A doe-eyed four-year-old came bounding out of the nearby wooden dollhouse and leaped onto the bench next to him. "This is Ellen," Dr. Sitkin said. "She's going to be a nephrologist when she grows up."

"I like kidneys," Ellen announced.

"I like kidneys, too," I said, "and it's a pleasure to meet you."

We chatted for ten minutes about my upcoming board exams, the new deck they were building in their home, and the receding dunes on the beach. When I'd finished my coffee, I bid them good-bye and hopped on my bike. I didn't often have a chance to socialize with my attendings. It felt nice. It felt like I was actually growing up.

∽Seventeen months later I was returning home from a two-week vacation in Israel. It was a chilly January morning and I was walking down Broadway on the Upper West Side. I had arrived only yesterday and I was still jet-lagged, but not jet-lagged enough to pass up a quarter-pound of Zabar's best lox.

My mind was tired and it wandered from the British Airways billboard to the posters advertising upcoming rock concerts at Madison Square Garden. I saw a missing person flyers posted on a street lamp for a young college student who had disappeared from a New Year's Eve party. Probably overdosed on drugs, I thought, and walked past it. Then the thought suddenly struck me—that flyer represented a person. And not only a person, it represented a family in emotional panic. That kid was somebody's son, somebody's baby. How could I just walk by? A block away was another lamppost with another flyer posted on it and I walked deliberately over to it. I was going to pay these poor souls their due. The white photocopied paper was affixed with tape on the top and bottom, but the corners flew loose in the wind. Suddenly I found myself staring at the face of Joseph Sitkin. "Missing," it said, "since Monday. Last seen wearing blue jeans and yellow parka." The photo showed his trademark curly hair spilling over the edges of his wire-rimmed glasses.

I felt my legs grow weak as I grabbed the lamppost for support. I was sure my vision had been mistaken. These missing flyers were always filled with distorted photos of strangers whose presence or absence could not affect my life. There must have been some mistake.

I pulled myself back up and forced my eyes to gaze upon the flyer again. The photocopied version of the picture blurred the details and one couldn't make out the sharp wit and ample intelligence that I knew permeated the lean features of his face, but it was Dr. Sitkin, or at least a representation of Dr. Sitkin. It was a disembodied reflection of the man I knew, not just because of the warped physical details of the picture, but because of his very presence on such a poster. I felt like I was looking through a photographic negative, and there was something discomfortingly unbalanced about seeing the opposite of presence. I was staring at his absence. How could Dr. Sitkin be missing?

I spotted an acquaintance on the street, someone not part of the medical field, and I pointed out the flyer, asking if she had heard about this. "Oh yes," she said. "It's been all over the news this week. His wife was on TV and everything."

How could I have been so out of touch with the news while I was in Israel?

I raced to the medical school library, where I knew that a week's worth of the *New York Times* would remain stashed on a shelf before being discarded. I flipped furiously through the pages of the back issues until I stumbled upon the headline, "Prominent Manhattan Doctor Missing from Upper West Side Apartment." I scanned the text desperately. "Dr. Joseph Sitkin was last seen Monday morning." "Always jogged in the early mornings." "Nothing missing from apartment." "No sign of foul play."

In the issue two days later there was another article entitled, "Missing Doctor Left Note on Computer." My heart pounded as I read on. "The letter on Dr. Sitkin's computer spoke of his despondency." Despondency? The man who always had a joke on hand? The man who marveled at his daughter's ability to fit all of her toes in her mouth? "Dr. Sitkin's long, rambling letter chronicled his increasing despair as well as his love for his wife and two daughters."

The newspapers crumpled in my hand and I crumpled in my seat. How could this have happened? Were there any signs? Could we have known? Or helped?

For the next week there was a palpable tension at the medical center. Rumors circulated that Dr. Sitkin had had a nervous breakdown and was recuperating somewhere anonymously. Someone said there was a report of a credit card purchase in East Hampton and that he must be out at their summer home.

On January 29th, two weeks from the date of his disappearance, a body washed ashore. "A badly decomposed body was found on the rocks," the *New York Times* read the next day, "under the Manhattan side of the George Washington Bridge, and the police tentatively identified it as that of Dr. Joseph Sitkin, a prominent Manhattan doctor who disappeared two weeks ago and left a note ..."

I closed my eyes from the headlines, unable to read on. How could it have felt, I agonized to myself, to stand on that bridge in the early chill of the morning and stare down at the Hudson River swirling below? How much must his heart have ached as his palm rested upon the frigid metal handrail? With how much despair must his legs have trembled as he eased his athletic limbs over the edge? How much anguish must he have possessed to combat the vertiginous assault of facing down the furious river?

I could only put my hand over my mouth and clamp my already closed eyes even further shut to block out the vision of his final moments. But I couldn't erase the internal vision of his pain and that of his wife, Julie. I shuddered at the thought of that icy moment of transition from her annoyance of his being late to her panic at his absence. The distraught days of unknowing, like a slowly cranked torture rack. The discovery of his letter, of the worst fears confirmed. And the baffling illogic of the world to render this comprehensible to two little girls.

The next day I found myself crammed in the downtown #1 train with the press of morning commuters. I slithered open my *New York Times* just a crack to peek at the news. I found myself at the obituaries and there it was: "Sitkin, Joseph, beloved husband of Julie, devoted father of Andrea and Ellen, dead at the age of thirty-nine. According to his wishes, the family has donated his body to the Microbiology Department at NYU Medical Center." It was suddenly so real, so final. I began to sniffle and swallow. And then the tears began to creep out. Someone offered me a seat and suddenly I began to cry unabashedly. The commuters looked on in helpless confusion. A woman asked me if I was feeling okay. I pointed to the obituary and said, "I knew him. That doctor from NYU who's been missing, I knew him. He was one of my teachers." And I bawled openly amid the embarrassed silence of the subway car.

I escaped from the subway and walked the remaining thirty blocks home. Thirty painful blocks. Thirty blocks of remembering the comatose alcoholic with the shofar by his side and the twelve pints of Ben & Jerry's ice cream for breakfast. Thirty blocks of remembering how

Dr. Sitkin encouraged Lauren's powerful song, and the way he always glanced at the Polaroid photo of Ms. Chen's baby taped to the railing of Bed 7. Thirty blocks of remembering how he made me laugh and how I actively struggled to dislike him but just couldn't. Thirty blocks of remembering the tough work and the extraordinary payoff of earning Dr. Sitkin's respect.

⁂Ours is a dangerous profession, I've often thought. There is the constant assault of physical and emotional challenges of taking care of patients that is layered upon the already difficult task of conducting our own lives. It is no wonder that so many of us become overwhelmed at times and need some intensive care. For every Dr. Sitkin who eventually declares his pain to the world, there are probably fifty others who suffer silently, for whom the anguish burns slowly and excruciatingly. The medical profession has little room or patience for hearing about this. These feelings often get expressed as bitter, abusive personalities, or drug and alcohol addictions.

The cliché says that doctors make the worst patients, that they are the last to seek treatment. We are always trying to help our patients get beyond their denial, but it seems that we use it most for ourselves. Is that the Faustian bargain we make when we enter the profession? I don't want to believe that is true, but for some it is apparently so.

CHAPTER FIFTEEN

Merced

For this is the end of examinations
For this is the beginning of testing
For Death will give the final examination
and everyone will pass

John Stone, *"Gaudeamus Igitur"*

"THIS IS A CASE OF A twenty-three-year-old Hispanic female, without significant past medical history, who presented to Bellevue Hospital complaining of a headache." The speaker droned on with the details of the case that I knew so well. I leaned back in my chair, anticipating and savoring the accolades that were going to come. After all, in a roundabout way, I'd made the diagnosis. I was the one who had the idea to send the Lyme test in the first place.

Mercedes had been to two other ERs before showing up at Bellevue three weeks ago. I was only doing sick call that day because Roger, one of the other residents, had twisted his knee playing volleyball. Mercedes was a classic aseptic meningitis, the kind that you'd send home with aspirin and some chicken soup, but the ER had decided to admit her to the hospital. Her CT scan was normal, and the spinal tap just showed a few lymphocytes, but the ER always overreacts. They gave her IV antibiotics even though there was no hint of the life-threatening bacterial meningitis.

One of the ER docs had scrawled something about "bizarre behavior" on the chart and had given her a stat dose of acyclovir. Another ridiculous ER maneuver; this patient had no signs of herpes encephalitis.

I'll admit that I was a little cocky that day. But I was just two months short of finishing residency and I knew a lot more medicine than those

ER guys. I chewed them out for admitting her and made a big show of canceling the acyclovir order.

When I met Mercedes on that first day, she was sleeping on a stretcher in a corner of the ER. I had to wake her up to take the history, but after a few shakes she was completely lucid. With her plump cheeks and wide brown eyes, she didn't even look seventeen, much less twenty-three. The sleeves of her pink sweatshirt were pushed up past her elbows. A gold cross with delicate filigree was partly obscured by the folds of the sweatshirt.

"Doctor, you have to believe me," she said, pulling herself up on the stretcher. "I've never been sick a day in my life. It's only this past month that I've been getting these headaches. They come almost every day and aspirin doesn't do anything. I came to the ER yesterday but they said, 'You got nothin' lady,' and just gave me a couple of Tylenols." Dark curls spilled over her pink shirt. They were mussed with a gentle just-woken-up look. While she spoke, one hand wove itself absentmindedly in and out of the locks.

"So, what made you come back today?" I asked.

"This headache, it didn't go away. And then my arm. It got all pins and needles for a few minutes. Just a couple of minutes, but now it's fine." Mercedes smiled slightly, and two tiny dimples flickered in her cheeks. "I guess they got tired of me complaining, so they decided to let me stay."

I did a thorough physical exam, spending extra time on the neurologic part. I checked every reflex I could think of: biceps, triceps, brachoradialis, patellar, plantar. I examined all twelve cranial nerves. Everything seemed normal. I tried to do all the obscure neurological tests I could remember from *Bates' Textbook of Physical Diagnosis,* but nothing seemed amiss. She was certainly not behaving bizarrely.

From talking to her, I learned that Mercedes was a single mother with two children aged three and four. She lived with her own mother, but still maintained a close relationship with the father of her children. She worked as a preschool teacher in upper Manhattan. She was born in Puerto Rico but since moving to the United States at age two, had never left the country.

I questioned her extensively about possible exposure to viruses or atypical organisms: travel to the countryside, recent illnesses, recent vaccinations, outbreaks of sickness at her preschool, HIV risk factors, contact with pets, poorly cooked fish or meat … all of which she denied.

Based on her history and physical exam, I concluded that she had garden-variety aseptic meningitis. The ER staff, with their usual sledgehammer approach to medical care, had overdone it with intravenous antibiotics and acyclovir. Mercedes didn't even need to stay in the hospital, but she'd already been officially admitted. The administrative folks would have a conniption if I sent a patient home just two hours after checking in.

Just to show the ER docs how real academic medicine was done, I wrote up an extensive admission note for Mercedes, detailing all the rare causes of aseptic meningitis listed in *Harrison's*. Paragraph after paragraph elucidated my clinical logic, a textbook example of orderly scientific thinking. And I printed neatly, so it would be easy for anyone perusing the chart to read.

There was an extra tube of Mercedes's cerebrospinal fluid sitting in my pocket, so I decided to send it for a couple of rare tests, including a Lyme titre. What the heck, I thought. This is a teaching institution. We're supposed to waste some money on exotic tests in order to learn. Besides, it would really impress the attending on rounds tomorrow, when I would blithely nod my head at each diagnosis he'd ask about.

Lyme? "Done."

Rickettsia? "Got it."

Sarcoid? "Covered."

Coxsackievirus? "Sent it."

Toxoplasmosis? "Already there."

Lupus? "Done."

The ER docs might just toss a heap of medications at anyone who walked in the door, but here in the Department of Medicine, we utilized our diagnostic acumen.

The next morning during rounds, just as I was dazzling the crowd with my erudite analysis of Mercedes's case, the nurses called me urgently to Mercedes's room. Mercedes was on the floor with her clothes off, hair askew, babbling incoherently. Her IV had been pulled out and her body was splattered with blood. Completely disoriented, she fought us vociferously as we tried to help her back to bed.

Thirty minutes later she was entirely back to normal—soft-spoken, polite, appropriately responsive to our questions, neatly groomed. She had no recollection of what had occurred and I was absolutely dumbfounded. What the hell had just happened?

Immediately I repeated a CT scan and spinal tap, but the results were no different than they'd been the day before. The neurologist felt Mercedes's behavior might have represented a seizure of the temporal lobe. The herpes virus has a predilection for the temporal lobe so this episode might have been a sign of herpes encephalitis. Regretting my earlier haughtiness toward the ER staff, I quietly restarted the acyclovir.

Mercedes was transferred to the neurology unit for management of herpes encephalitis, and I was transferred off the ward when Roger's knee got better. I was happy to get back to my cushy dermatology elective.

A week later, still smarting from missing the herpes encephalitis diagnosis, I tracked down the intern to see how Mercedes was doing. "Hey, did you hear the news?" he asked. "That herpes encephalitis patient really had Lyme disease. The test just came back positive yesterday."

Lyme disease? The Lyme test I that I had sent came back positive? I was exhilarated. This would be the most fascinating diagnosis on the medical wards. Who would have suspected that a New York City dweller would have a disease carried by deer ticks in the forest. But hey, I did a careful diagnostic evaluation of the patient, and my thoroughness paid off.

Soon everybody was talking about the case of Lyme meningitis in our inner-city hospital. The head of my residency program became interested in the case and suggested I plan a seminar on Lyme disease. I set about obtaining all the details of Mercedes's case and searched the medical literature for current articles on Lyme disease.

Meanwhile, Mercedes was started on the appropriate medication for Lyme. She'd been discharged home and was finishing her three-week course of antibiotics with daily shots in the clinic.

Today the case was being presented at neurology grand rounds. I wasn't a participant in this particular conference, but I didn't care. I sat back in my chair and listened to speaker after speaker comment on the "incredible diagnosis" that had been made. My bulging "Mercedes/Lyme" folder sat on my lap as I took mental notes, preparing for my own presentation in the Department of Medicine two weeks from now.

Residency would be over at the end of next month. I had been here for ten years, from the beginning of medical school, through my PhD, and then my residency. Ten years of medical training! But now it was truly paying off. Ten years of the scientific approach to medicine had prepared me for this case. Ten years of emphasis on careful analysis of data—whether of receptor binding assays in the lab, or signs and symptoms in a patient—had taught me how to establish a hypothesis and come to a logical conclusion. This was the academic way that ensured the highest quality medical care. Our attendings were always pointing out medical disasters that occurred "out in the community" with doctors who were not academic physicians. Doctors who didn't keep up with the latest medical journals. Doctors who, without diligent and thoughtful analysis, ordered any old test or prescribed any fancy packaged medicine marketed by the pharmaceutical companies.

Mercedes was lucky to have come to an academic medical center rather than to a community hospital, where her diagnosis would have been missed entirely. Just like Mr. Wiszhinsky on my first day at Bellevue as a medical student. His life was saved by his good fortune of coming to Bellevue.

What a fantastic case for my residency training to culminate with. I could use this as an illustrative diagnostic case for my students of the future. Maybe I would submit this to the *New England Journal of Medicine*.

Someone had invited Mercedes to the conference, and she sat in the back listening quietly. I watched her from my vantage point in the corner. She looked wonderful on that Friday afternoon–no hint of the illness that caused that bizarre episode on her second hospital day. I shook her hand heartily and congratulated her on her recovery. Her hand was warm and plump, and her handshake reassuringly healthy.

Monday morning I joined our new team in the ICU. This was my last month of residency and I was going to spend it in the ICU. There was a crackle in the air of all the different machines breathing life into our critically ill patients. We rounded on all of our new patients as a tightly honed team, talking in easy jargon with no need to translate for anyone. At each bedside was a computer that was loaded with data for each patient. We raced each other to calculate arterial-alveolar gradients and oxygen extraction ratios. We reeled off ventilator management strategies, debating the relative values of positive end-expiratory pressure versus continuous positive airway pressure. I marveled at how easy it all was. As an intern, or even a second-year resident, the ICU was a terrifying place, especially the first day. But now I took it all in stride. Just another twelve sick patients on ventilators with arterial lines and Swans. Let 'em crash, let 'em code. . . . I knew I could handle it. That's what ten years of Bellevue training does for you. Once you've been in the belly of the beast, nothing fazes you.

That evening I was home alone, gathering my thoughts about my new set of patients. It was only Monday, but I knew it was going to be an exciting month. Residency was going to end in style. Our team was going to get this ICU into top shape.

But the old guy in Bed 5 who'd stroked out last month—left side not moving, already demented from Alzheimer's. I wasn't sure if his ventilator settings were optimized; his peak pressures had been fluctuating. I was sure I could do better. Why wait until tomorrow if I could keep that patient one step ahead? If I could get the latest blood gas results now, I could make the adjustments over the phone and then see his progress before rounds in the morning. I propped my feet up on my couch and tore open a bag of chili-and-lime tortilla chips. One hand dialed the phone while the other plunged into the bag. This was going to be a great month.

Instead of the clerk who usually answered the phone, George, one of the other residents, happened to answer. We chatted for a while about how much fun the ICU was and what a great way it was to end residency. We discussed the ventilator management of Bed 5 and agreed to lower the flow rate but increase the tidal volume. I asked how his first night on call was going.

"What a night," George said. "We've been incredibly busy. One cardiac arrest, one septic shock. But my third admission is the most interesting. It's a good one. You ain't never seen this before."

"Really," I said, pulling out a handful of red, powdery chips. "What did you get?"

"It's a surprise. Something rare. You'll see on tomorrow's rounds."

"Give me a hint," I said between chomps of chips. "I covered for you on your anniversary last March. You owe me one."

I pestered him some more, and then he finally relented. In a conspiratorially low voice, to tantalize my curiosity he said, "Read up on Lyme meningitis for rounds tomorrow."

The chips and chili turned to sawdust in my mouth. I blinked a few times, my brain slow to react. "That's strange," I said, the words like cardboard wading through the sawdust. "I just had a case of Lyme meningitis three weeks ago." I could feel the muscles in my neck tightening. My throat began to constrict. Please God, don't let it be the same person. Don't let it be Mercedes.

"Yep, that's the one," George said.

Mercedes? In the ICU? I became frantic for air. I had just seen her on Friday and she was fine. How could she be in the ICU on Monday? I ground the sticky plastic of the telephone into my ear, struggling to absorb the story that was being transmitted.

On Saturday, George told me, Mercedes had experienced another headache. On Sunday her headache worsened so she came to the ER.

Nothing was found on physical exam and she was sent home with a diagnosis of "post-meningitic headache," a frequent phenomenon.

On Monday, this afternoon, she complained of the "worst headache of her life," accompanied by nausea and vomiting. She returned to the ER and this time she was admitted to the hospital. The doctors who spoke with her said she was able to give a coherent history of her recent treatment, and again had a perfectly normal neurological exam. Nonetheless, they sent her for a CT scan of her head.

The CT scan lasted about fifteen minutes. When the technician went to help her out of the scanner, he found her unresponsive. A code was called, but by the time the code team arrived her pupils were already fixed and dilated: a sign of irreversible brain swelling. She was brought to the ICU, where a hole was drilled in her skull in an attempt to relieve the pressure, but it was too late.

Steroids were given to decrease the inflammation. Antibiotics of every stripe were administered. Various maneuvers to lower her intracranial pressure were attempted—artificially increasing her breathing rate, angling the bed to keep her head above her feet, infusing massive doses of osmotic diuretics—but none worked. Now she lay in Bed 10 of the ICU, her breathing maintained by a ventilator . . . brain dead.

Tests for tuberculosis, lupus, syphilis, vasculitis, and other inflammatory diseases were performed and all were negative.

"Could this all be from the Lyme?" I stammered, the tortilla crumbs petrifying my tongue.

"Nah," George replied. "We sent another Lyme titre and it came back negative. This ain't Lyme."

The Lyme test was negative?

"Yeah, the first Lyme was a false positive," George said. His voice faded for a minute as he told one of the nurses to suction Bed 4.

How could this whole thing have happened? How could a young woman, whom we had presumably cured, who had been so alive and healthy three days ago, be brain dead now?

I stormed back and forth in the two rooms of my apartment, crashing up against the infernally cramped dimensions that pass for living space in Manhattan. I called a pulmonologist that I knew and paged two of my residency colleagues but the case didn't make any sense to them. I tore my textbooks off the shelves, ripping through the indices for answers. I upended the contents of my "Mercedes/Lyme" folder, scouring the fine print in the scientific papers, hurling them aside when they proved useless.

Lyme in the inner city? How could I have been such an idiot to believe those results? A false positive—how could I have been so stupid?

This could not be happening. This Mercedes could not be the same as the Friday Mercedes, who'd smiled at me when I shook her hand. The Friday Mercedes was real. This Monday Mercedes was just a case report over the phone. It couldn't be real.

Should I go over to Bellevue to see? Should I verify in person what I'd been hearing over the phone? But the neurosurgeons were already there and the head of the infectious disease unit had personally examined Mercedes. She was already receiving the best nursing and medical care available. In reality, I knew that there was nothing I could add. Everything would still be the same on morning rounds a few hours from now. Anyway, I might be overstepping my bounds if I went in at this late hour, somehow insinuating that George's care was inadequate. Besides, once the pupils are fixed and dilated, everyone knows that there is nothing else to do.

It was now two A.M. I couldn't sit still and I'd run out of friends who I could call at that hour. I tried to convince myself that it would be for the greater good of all my patients if I just calmed down and got a good night of sleep so I could function in the morning. But my hands wouldn't stop shivering and I had already eaten all the chocolate I could unearth in my apartment.

I pulled on an old pair of scrubs and set off down First Avenue. The street was quiet—even the homeless had gone off somewhere to sleep. The gloomy brick behemoths of the old Bellevue buildings cast spooky shadows in the moonlight. The decaying TB sanatorium and mental hospital menaced from behind tall cast-iron gates. The dusky ivy on the brick buildings gave the walls a moist, velvety appearance. The scalloped columns in the abandoned courtyard poked eerily out of the ground like portals into some dark netherworld. I made my way through the midnight heaviness, my feet only vaguely aware of the sidewalk beneath them. From the faint lights in the garden I could just see the dark shadows that were the birdbath and fountain.

But inside the hospital building it was brightly lit. I squinted at the shock of light as I walked down the long white hallways, past the closed coffee shop, past the darkened candy store, past the sleepy security guard. I felt blurry from the incongruity of it all—the Mercedes that I had seen on Friday had disappeared and a new one had been substituted. How could normal hospital life go on when such unearthly alchemy was occurring in its midst?

I tiptoed into the ICU. From the doorway I saw George facing Mercedes's family and friends who were gathered around Bed 10. I edged in closer, but the bed was obscured by the people standing around it. George was trying vainly to explain the finality of the situation. Mercedes's mother and two sisters were sobbing openly. Her brother stood motionless, his eyes occasionally quivering within his otherwise frozen expression of bewilderment. Some friends clustered around the sisters, hugging them and weeping.

I hovered by the supply cart, forcibly swallowing against the sticky walls of my throat. In the surreal penumbra of the ICU, the family blended into a landscape of backs, with shadowed peaks and dips surrounding a central canyon. The fluorescent lights from the bed arose within their mountainous midst and glinted up off their faces, creating awkward silhouettes and oddly sculpted ravines. I crept closer to the rocky human formation, hoping that no one would notice me. The light within drew me forward with a queasy gravitation. I had to see what was inside. The air seemed to thin out as I drew closer and I had to work harder to breathe. As I neared the bed my stomach rebelled and I placed a hand on it to keep it down. A rivulet of yellowish-green light seeped from between the mother and one of the cousins. I squinted into the crack of light to see what lay in Bed 10.

It was Mercedes, the one that I knew.

It was the same Friday Mercedes, with luminous cheeks and luxurious black hair cascading on the pillow. Her eyelids were softly closed and the dark lashes rested in delicate parallel lines upon her olive cheeks. Her gold filigree cross floated along the plump, unblemished skin of her neck. Her respirations were calm and even, thanks to the ventilator. Aside from the breathing tube, she looked like a beautiful, healthy woman who was only sleeping.

From the electronic monitors overhead, though, a different story was evident. The red line indicating the pressure inside of Mercedes's head was undulating menacingly at the edge of the screen, nearly off the scale entirely. Despite all of the medical interventions, her brain was swelling inside the solid walls of her skull. A pressure chamber was roiling inside those unforgiving cranial bones, driving the base of her brain out the bottom of her skull. The respiratory center of her brain had already been trampled by the relentless onslaught. The cardiac center would soon follow.

How could this be my Friday Mercedes?

The brother noticed me standing behind the crowd and then the whole family turned to me. Nobody said anything, but I could feel the desperation of their eyes, those longing eyes, beseeching me to offer them something that hadn't yet been tried. But I was still trying to reconcile my own reality. I was still trying to convince myself that this was the same Mercedes I'd seen on Friday. That this beautiful, sleeping woman was the same woman we'd so triumphantly diagnosed with Lyme disease only three weeks ago.

And now brain dead. All because I'd sent that damn Lyme test.

Usually when I've had to explain to a family that a patient is dying, the patient graciously assists me by looking the part. They are pale or emaciated, or in pain, or struggling for breath: they look like death. But Mercedes refused to play along. Serenely she lay, as beautiful as she'd been three days ago: no scars from repeated IVs and blood draws, no skin ulcers from prolonged immobility, no dull coating of the skin from weeks of not seeing the sun. No, she looked steadfastly alive.

But she was dead. Brain dead is dead. There is no gray area in brain death. Mercedes's "lifefulness" was just an illusion granted by the ventilator and the short duration of her condition. In a day or two her body would swell up and her skin would grow dusky. The cardiac center of her brain would be smothered by the persistent intracranial swelling and her heart would finally give out. Then Mercedes would look like the death that we knew and our senses trusted.

The hospital chaplain arrived. He was a rotund, balding, Catholic priest whom I had seen around the hospital but never met. A Bellevue ID card and a wooden crucifix dangled from his neck. They settled on the flare of his belly, competing with each other for prominence as he moved about. He slowly made his way around the bed, touching each family member, offering tissues, murmuring softly. I could see each person's body relax ever so slightly at his touch. With his pudgy white hands he seemed to spread soft dapples of comfort. His job looked so much more palatable than mine. How simple just to be the bearer of solace.

He glanced at me from across the bed where he was standing with one of the sisters and he must have seen a tear welling up in my eye. He circled back to where I stood and silently reached out his arm, resting it upon my shoulder. The gentle weight settled onto my shoulder blades. It absorbed into the strain of my back, melting the muscles that were clenching and smothering me. My stethoscope twisted off my neck onto the floor as I leaned into his black tunic and began to cry. His arms circled around me like the comforting arms of Angeline Burton after I'd been stuck by a needle during her hysterectomy. And my body reacted similarly to that touch, unraveling and letting go. I collapsed deeper into his chest, sobbing and sobbing. The family stared with quiet amazement as I cried uncontrollably in the arms of a strange priest. One of the sisters left Mercedes's side and came to me. She stroked my back, her fingers running along my hair.

I cried for Mercedes. I cried for her family and her two little children. I cried for Eileen O'Neil and her mother and aunt, and her two sons. I cried for Raphael Herlan and his lover John. I cried for Margaret Whitney in her enduring coma and her daughter, Sandra, with her endless vigil. I cried for Dr. Schwartz and his painful months of denial. I cried for Mr. Teitelbaum and his death among strangers. And I cried for my Josh.

I cried for the death of my belief that intellect conquers all.

When I ran out of tears and stamina, I said quiet, embarrassed good-byes to Mercedes's family. The older sister handed me my stethoscope. She took my hand, looked me straight in the eye, and said "Thank you" with such sincerity that I felt guilty. Her sister was dying and instead of me comforting her, she was offering comfort to me.

I stumbled out of Bellevue in a daze. It was raining and I didn't have an umbrella. Dawn hadn't yet risen over the East River, but the air was lighter. I was exhausted, but felt strangely relieved. That uncontrollable nervous energy had finally abated and the drenching rain felt cleansing.

I stayed up the rest of the night and wrote down as much about Mercedes as I could remember. For the first time in my ten years of medical training, sleep did not interest me.

Four weeks later I completed my internal medicine residency. My ten years at Bellevue had finally ended. There was little pomp as I limped out of the ICU all alone on a rainy Sunday morning after my final thirty-six-hour shift. Bed 2 was coding, but somebody else was taking care of it.

My body drooped with exhaustion, its muscles depleted and quivering from the mere effort of walking. And my soul felt drained, aching for rest. I couldn't think beyond unloading these 206 bones into a soft, warm, horizontal bed. I couldn't fathom opening a newspaper tomorrow, much less starting a fellowship or a job, like most of my colleagues were doing. I needed repose.

I knew that I had to get out of Bellevue, even if for just a little while—away from residency, away from training, away from death. I didn't know exactly what I wanted to do, but I knew I had to do something different. I could feel a whispered embrace from Josh. He continued to remind me, with both his love and his loss, that I had to live.

There would always be decades of medicine awaiting me, but there might never be another time to slip away, to uncurl, to open up. I signed up with a *locum tenens* agency, which would allow me to do short-term medical jobs anywhere in the country—after a two-month summer break, of course. I planned to work only one month at a time, and then travel as far as the money would take me. I wanted to go to Central America to see the native countries of so many of my patients at Bellevue. I wanted to learn the language that had prevented me from communicating with them. And I had to write down my stories from Bellevue.

I purchased a laptop computer that could fit into my backpack. I stocked up on as many novels as I could carry and canceled my subscription to the *New England Journal of Medicine.*

But Mercedes continued to haunt me. For the next two years, between my travels and my locums assignments, I cornered every neuropathologist who could spare a moment to hear her story. I faxed her case history to experts at different medical centers and hounded them with phone calls, but no one had an answer for me. Mercedes's autopsy was "unrevealing" and every test was negative or "nondiagnostic." The medical examiner eventually signed the case out as "unknown etiology."

Something had killed Mercedes, why couldn't we figure it out? How come, with all of our CT scans, intracranial monitors, immunologic assays, and third-generation antibiotics, a young healthy woman could walk into the hospital with a headache and then be dead within hours? I may as well have applied amulets and recited incantations. Ten years of training, of memorizing complex formulas, of cramming differential diagnoses—blithely squelched by some anonymous microbe. None of my professors had ever prepared me for this. None of my textbooks had ever talked about this. None of the diagnostic algorithms that we discussed on rounds had ever taken this into account. None of the multiple choice questions on our board exams ever offered this as a possible answer. There was no academic medical subspecialty dedicated to this.

What will Mercedes's children think of the medical profession, I wondered. Their mother, of whom they'll have only dim recollections, had died mysteriously and the doctors never knew why. I wanted to go to them and apologize for our shortcomings, our limited intellect, our inadequate tools, the false pride that led us down the wrong path, our utter failure. But they are in their own world, being raised by a loving, extended family.

And while I was intellectually frustrated, I felt strangely emotionally complete. That night in the ICU with Mercedes was excruciatingly painful, but it was also perhaps my most authentic experience as a doctor. Something was sad. And I cried. Simple logic, but so rarely adhered to in the high-octane world of academic medicine. Standing in the ICU, the chaplain's arms around me, surrounded by Mercedes's family, I felt like a person. Not like a physician or a scientist or an emissary from the world of rational logic, but just a person. Like each of the other persons who were locked in that tight circle around Bed 10. There was a strength in that circle that I'd never felt from my colleagues or my professors. A strength that allowed me to release the tense determination for intellectual mastery that had so supported me as a doctor. After years of honing those muscles, it was a deliriously aching relief to let them go.

And it didn't turn me away from medicine; it enticed me. I did need a break, but I knew that I would come back. I still wanted to learn more and become a smarter doctor, but I also wanted to be in this world populated with living, breathing, feeling people. I wanted to be in this sacred zone that was alive with real feelings, theirs and mine. I still didn't know why I had initially entered the field of medicine ten years ago, but I now knew why I wanted to stay.

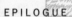

Possessing Her Words

SEVEN DAYS WE WAITED for Adrienne Berneau.

Seven days we held her words, knowing they might be her last. We had promised her we'd only allow her one week on the ventilator. If she didn't improve, and if it became clear that her cancer was winning, we'd unplug it. We'd promised her.

✎Waiting and holding—two of the burdens of medicine. Much has been written of the physical burdens of medical training, and there are many. And indeed these were the ones I had feared the most as I began medical school. How would I manage without sleep? Could I possibly memorize those millions of diseases? How would I pass all the medical boards? Those did turn out to be grueling tasks, but it seemed that if I just pushed myself hard enough, they could be surmounted.

But as I moved along from medical student to intern to resident to attending, the challenges became far more profoundly taxing, not just to address, but even to name.

Waiting. Holding. These were not in the index of *Harrison's Textbook of Internal Medicine*.

Waiting is something physicians do not do well. We demand rapid results—from our diagnostic tests, from our patients and, most mercilessly, from ourselves. We are not patient with ourselves. We rarely permit ourselves to wait in solitude, to allow the poetic subtleties and convoluted irrationalities of patient care to sink deep within us. We may know that we are frustrated, or perhaps gratified, by a particular encounter, but we seldom offer ourselves the time and space to understand why.

Contrary to the stereotype, doctors do not lack for emotions. The medical student is too embarrassed to ask a patient to undress for a physical exam. The intern is sweating and cursing because the IV won't go in on the seventh try and she hasn't seen sunshine in three days. The resident is angry at the cocaine addict whose refusal of a CT scan will make him stay late again and miss, once again, putting his kids to bed. The attending is nervous on rounds because he's a bit "rusty" with his inpatient skills and the residents might get wind of his ignorance.

Emotions punctuate the speech and actions of all characters in this drama, but most doctors are not aware of the myriad levels of emotional resonance, other than that they feel annoyed and want to get the hell out of the hospital as quickly as possible. It is both awkward and daunting to stop and wait. If we slow down and see where these feelings redound, we risk becoming too vulnerable. And so we walk and talk with a feverish clip to keep the reflective silence at bay.

The seven days that Adrienne Berneau forced us to wait was a terrifying and awe-inspiring time. When the four of us left her room, we were shaken to the bone. None of our ready-to-wear parlances could stand up to that moment. We had no choice but to be still and wait— to let the atmosphere of that room worm its way downward and inward, through to our very marrows. And the real burden, the real challenge, of being a physician became manifest.

We held her words within us, not knowing if these would be her last. Like cupping a butterfly in one's palms, there was the physical tension of clenched fingers in a disconcerting balance against the requisite gentleness to protect the tender treasure. Physicians do much holding, but are rarely conscious of the action or what it might portend. We take histories from patients, write them down on paper, recite them on rounds, sometimes relate them to friends over a beer as good "war stories," but we rarely take time to contemplate this act of history-taking. We are holding the patient's story—their words, their voices, their facial expressions, their fears, their needs, their trust—cupped in our palms. When we trudge home at night and feel the cricks straining across our shoulders, we usually ascribe it to the many hours we have just spent on our feet. And that is part of it, but another part is the weight of balancing so many patients' stories within us.

I do not recall anyone talking about this particular type of strain during my residency training. We all complained about the hours and the fatigue and the noncompliant patients and the incompetent nurses and the useless attendings, but rarely about the painful weight of so much holding. Occasionally we were required to attend "touchy-feely" rounds in which we were supposed to reveal our inner stresses to a well-meaning social worker, but those usually degenerated into complaining sessions. And so we walked around with piercing exhaustion, but never much explored the components of it beyond the ever-present sleeplessness.

When I started this book, my desire was to get down all the stories I'd acquired from Bellevue, the ones I'd been telling friends and family about over the years. The ones that usually began with, "You'll never believe what happened to me today ..." But as the stories laid themselves out, it was the relationship to those stories that rose to the forefront. The stresses of residency began to unfold in layers far more intricate than mere fatigue. Once I slowed myself down and re-experienced the tension of holding all those stories, of waiting for all the feelings to percolate down from the unruly muck into something more understandable, the book began to change. I started to understand how complex the act of becoming a doctor really was.

And although many of the stories revolve around gravely ill patients who die in stark and painful fashion, these don't completely illustrate the full spectrum of being a doctor. It is sometimes in the most mundane clinical encounters, the ones that don't lend themselves to a dramatic retelling, that medicine is most uplifting. The smile on the patient's face upon hearing that her cholesterol has come down, the gratitude from the patient when you prescribe a three-month supply of pills instead of a one-month supply, the triumph of finding a Bengali interpreter just when you need one—these are but splinters of satisfaction, but they are evermore common than the tormented deaths of the ICU. And these splinters, when coalesced, form a potent girder of fulfillment beneath me.

It is axiomatic that many patients die—this is medicine after all and not accounting—but I do not find medicine to be a depressing field. Sad at times, yes, but depressing no. The human connections made with these patients, indeed inspired by them, is compelling. It is this that makes it possible, and even joyous, to continue.

℘When I left Mme. Berneau's bedside that evening, I wanted so much to be home quickly, to escape the tension. But as I strode out of Bellevue, the garden beckoned. The wooden benches and meandering walks called to me to slow down. The multitiered fountain was now flowing with water, lovingly restored recently by the auxiliary association. The bubbling sound, though probably not significant decibel-wise, somehow seemed able to neutralize much of the dissonant twentieth-century sounds pressing in from beyond the slender cast-iron fencing. The three-legged birdbath was sitting in its quiet patch of grass and I walked over. To my surprise, I discovered that it had four legs, not three; all these years I'd been mistaken. The delightful symmetry of the legs was such that when viewed from almost any angle, the fourth leg was always playfully hidden by its identical opposite, giving the illusion of three legs. And when I took a closer look, I discovered that although pigeons congregated there freely, it was not, in fact, a birdbath at all, but an old sundial. Another thing I'd missed all these years. The round face of the clock was set into an elongated marble diamond, which was itself set into the circular tabletop. When viewed from the side, it appeared almost as a contemplating eye. The shadow stick for telling time was gone, so the numbers of the sundial lay quiet and unused. I peered closer at the numbers and realized that the numbers at the bottom of the dial were not numbers, but letters. Yet another surprise. They were crammed tightly together but I was able to decipher the engraving. "Grow old along with me, the best is yet to be"—a quote from Robert Browning.

One never knows, I thought to myself, where poetry will turn up in one's life. It took ten years for me to stumble upon this tiny gift even though I'd passed by it nearly every day. What other flashes of poetry from the pedestrian have I missed over these years? I could feel Josh's gentle reminders whispering against my skin, reminding me to attend to the rhythms and metre of my everyday surroundings.

For decades, I'd pressed ahead in school and in medical training without much thought for the pace or the outcome. The loss of Josh during internship abruptly drained much of the brightness from the palette with which I'd viewed my future. Passing the boards, vying for a competitive fellowship, landing a choice scholarship—suddenly these goals lost their complexity of hue and with that, their patent urgency. An unsettled feeling—a mix of aching sorrow for Josh and a muddled sense of my overall purpose—began to worm its way through my body, never quite articulating how I should be changing, but gnawing at me, always gnawing, that something was now different.

By the end of residency, this inchoate drive impelled me to take a break from academic medicine. Traveling, reading, writing, thinking—these were things I hadn't had much time for during residency. I always knew I would return to Bellevue because I couldn't imagine practicing medicine anyplace else. When I finally did return several years later, a New York City hiring freeze permitted me to take on only a part-time faculty position. Writing began as a hobby for these serendipitous days off, but gradually expanded. These literary pursuits grew to fill my time, intertwining with my medical pursuits, sharpening that amorphous urge that had been gnawing at me since internship. I read my *Poets and Writers* with as much conviction as I did my *New England Journal of Medicine.* I divided my "continuing education" days between writing conferences and medical conferences. My social circle grew to encompass as many writers as doctors. Within four years, I found myself creating a literary jounal within Bellevue Hospital. The *Bellevue Literary Review* began as an idea to highlight medical student writings, but quickly grew to a national literary journal focused on the human condition as viewed through the prism of health and healing, illness and disease. Writers from diverse backgrounds contributed work, and suddenly I was editor in chief of a substantial literary journal.

The *Bellevue Literary Review* eventually required as much of my time as did patient care. My days became a blend of medical care and editorial review, discussions with physicians and with poets, critical appraisal of scientific papers and fiction manuscripts. If my beeper went off, it could just as easily be the emergency room as our publisher.

I never would have predicted this when I started my medical training, armed with a PhD in biochemistry, ready to translate the sturdy scientific principles directly into patient care. I've never lost the scientist in me—it still keeps me highly skeptical when I read of new medical innovations or new poetic structures—but it has blended comfortably into my current amalgam of medicine, writing, and editing. It is here, at the juncture of the medical and literary worlds, that I finally feel settled into my own skin. I would never give up medicine to be a full-time writer, and I could never give up writing to advance my career in medicine. It is as it should be.

✐Mme. Berneau remained in Bed 9 in the ICU. Because the sedatives were dropping her blood pressure dangerously, they had to be discontinued, and so I was unable to keep my promise that she would sleep for the entire seven days. She was awake but silent; the plastic tube in her throat had rendered her voiceless. She tried to gesture in response to my questions, but the IV line, arterial line, blood pressure cuff, pulse oximeter all shackled to her slender arms made her movements ungainly and imprecise.

The bronchoscopy and the CT scan were nondiagnostic. As happens so often in medicine, the burning question was never resolved. For all those days of waiting, we were never able to make a definitive diagnosis of infection versus recurring cancer. But we rooted for the microbes and continued to feed the "big-gun" antibiotics into her veins. Gradually, her oxygenation improved and her chest X-ray began to clear. Late Saturday night, on her fifth day of intubation, Adrienne Berneau yanked the tube out her throat and set herself free. There was no going back.

But she breathed on her own and it became clear in hindsight that she'd had an infection. Antibiotics—the wonder drugs of the twentieth century—had done their thing. Sunday morning was my last day as the attending on the wards for that month. I stopped by Bed 9 of the ICU and spoke with Mme. Berneau. There was no sweeter music than that silvery Parisian accent floating into my ears, lilting down my throat, caressing gently into my heart, and sweeping away that burden chafing in my soul. I would not have to be the bearer of Adrienne Berneau's final words on this earth.

We chatted about marvelously mundane things like the early spring weather and the decidedly un-French hospital food. Our words lofted between us with the casual air of an everyday miracle. Like a balloon tapped back and forth by sun-drenched fingertips, they bounced from her soul to mine and back again. The arc of our words shimmered in the air and her history settled softly into mine.

Acknowledgments

Benjy Akman thought he got off easy by marrying me post-residency, but instead found himself married into the process of writing a book, and probably still isn't sure if he got the better deal. Benjy has been my chief advocate, editor, reader, cheerleader, and computer fixer; I could never have done it without him. My writing teachers, Maureen Brady and Bill Black, were instrumental in shaping these stories. I also want to thank my writing buddies—Thomas Estler, Charlie Sahner, Marlene Lee—who patiently read endless iterations of these chapters, while asking only for cheese and crackers in return, and an occasional bit of whitefish salad.

Acknowledgment is made to the following publications in which versions of these writings appeared: *Best American Essays 2002* ("Merced"); *The Missouri Review* ("Merced," "M & M"); *Fourth Genre* ("Positive"); *Riverteeth* ("Stuck"); *New York Stories* ("Change of Heart"); *New Delta Review* ("July 1st"); *Cimarron Review* ("In Charge"); *Jabberwock Review* ("The Burden of Knowledge"); *New Millennium Writings* ("Time of Death: 3:27 A.M."); *Asphodel* ("Finding the Person"); *Under the Sun* ("Possessing Her Words"); and *Night Rally* ("AA Battery").

I am indebted to Helene Atwan, my editor at Beacon, whose clarity and optimism nudged this book to its final stages in a remarkably painless manner. With a few deft strokes of her red pen—and an occasional hack—she turned an unwieldy manuscript into a finished book. Her initial phone call to me, as I stood on the 16-East ward in Bellevue Hospital with thirty patients yet to see, perfectly captured the essence of doctoring and writing.

∽And of course I must thank my sweet daughter, Naava, who not only taught me how to breastfeed and edit at the same time, but provided an endless stream of love to keep my sights and priorities steady.